ISBN-13:
978-1533120434

ISBN-10:
1533120439

Dedication

This book is dedicated to you who knew how to prepare food and forgot, or was never taught; and to those of you who have not found the time to care for yourselves.
May this book in some way inspire you.

Thank You

To Julie Gissel who through the years, tried my food and encouraged me to share my ideas.
To Joan Riemer who taught me to write, to cook and to expand my horizons.
To Katie Rogers who helped me organize this project.
To Roxann Pope who brought beauty to this book.

Prologue

I entered acupuncture school because I wanted to learn how to use herbs to get a person well and keep her well. I was, and still am, under the opinion that it is acceptable to never be sick.

My mother took care of us as we were growing up. Her beginning health profession was nursing. From nursing, she expanded into Naturopathic Medicine which led her to Oriental Medicine.

From her I learned the importance of food; and that the type of food we ingest can create a harmonious and calm body, or riddle it with mucus and pain. Diet is the cornerstone of health as I define it. For myself or for my patients, I begin with food to balance and heal, and if something still needs mending, I use other modalities.

During my 25 years as an Acupuncturist, I have found that diet plans, beneficial or deleterious, play a key role in whether a patient gets well or not.

Food benefits your body. It keeps all the parts working as a whole unit.

If you eat the foods that support your strong qualities and that also strengthen your weak parts, you will add to your wellness.

The reverse is also true. If you eat foods that naturally thicken fluids when you have a cough or head cold, you will likely be sick for a longer period of time than what was really necessary.

Having a basic understanding of how food acts in your body will help you to put together foods that will taste good and help you to feel good.

Most of my patients do not lack for animal products in their diet. In fact, some of their diets are composed almost exclusively of animal products and grain or fruit. Vegetables and legumes rarely are seen; and if they are, they are in very small quantities.

When I mention a diet change, the usual response is either "I do not cook", or "do you have any recipes?"

The purpose of this book is to pass on my approach on food preparation and give some insights on how to use certain plant-based foods.

Since animal products are abundantly discussed in other books and video programs, I will let those products help you in all things concerning animal.

This book will re-introduce you to plant-based foods and how to use them creatively so that the produce section of the grocery store becomes an exciting place in which each vegetable gives you an idea for a potential meal.

After reading this book, you will be able to develop your own style of cooking that incorporates an approach to creating balanced meals.

Your meal preparation time will be short and not require hours of standing in the kitchen. Most of the recipes are based on a large serving for one person if you are hungry or two servings for company or leftovers for a second meal.

It is time to reintroduce you to your kitchen. You may not have used it much in the last few years, and that is all right. By the end of this book, your kitchen and you will be working together to bring you joy and health.

Contents

Chapter One
The Road to Now

Becoming Vegetarian

I am the youngest of five children. My home is Southern California, the place for sunshine all year long. It also is the place for fresh vegetables all year long.

I grew up with three sisters who could cook and/or bake. In those days, schedules were as busy as they are today, so that left very little room for me in the kitchen. My main job was clean up.

Our meals reflected the tradition of animal protein, salad, cooked vegetable and a starch. **My parents were health conscious.** Early on, my mother studied the effects of food on the body.

When my father got a little pudgy, he changed his diet to follow the guidelines of Carlton Fredricks *Inches Off Diet*. He successfully slimmed down.

On the other hand, my mother noticed a difference in how she felt when she ate animal flesh and when she did not. She found she felt better without much meat. That was when the diet of the family shifted to more lacto-ovo vegetarian meals. Cheese, eggs, nuts and beans replaced the animal flesh at our meals. Mostly.

We were not strict vegetarians. We ate vegetarian at home and indulged in animal flesh, if desired, when we ate out which was not more than once a week.

We ate Chinese food regularly. We generally made it at home but there was also a Chinese restaurant we went to across the alley from our house. We would each order our favorite dish. For the sister who had not developed a taste for Chinese food, she ordered a hamburger.

Fried Rice

1 cup cooked rice, best cold
1 ½ teaspoons soy sauce
1 ½ teaspoons water
1 egg, beaten
2 Tablespoons green onions, chopped
2 Tablespoons Earth Balance or butter
1 stalk celery, chopped

Heat a large frying pan over medium high heat. Add rice. Stir for 8 minutes to prevent sticking. Mix eggs into rice and stir briefly. Stir in onions, celery, soy sauce and water. Serve warm.

Chinese Broccoli

2 cups broccoli, cut into small florets
1 Tablespoons peanut oil
1 Tablespoons soy sauce
1 teaspoons ginger, grated
1 teaspoons agave nectar
2 Tablespoons hot water

In a small bowl, mix together soy sauce, ginger and agave nectar. Set aside.

Heat a wok or skillet over medium high heat. Add oil and broccoli and cook for 5 minutes. Stir soy sauce mixture into the broccoli mix well. Add hot water and cover pan. Cook for 2 minutes. Serve warm.

Besides animal flesh, we generally avoided white sugar, white flour and cow's milk. We used to drink homemade chocolate milk at dinner but that went by the wayside. Our options for liquids were water, diluted juice or Good Earth Tea. Coffee was limited to special occasions like dining out.

Attitude

During my teens we entertained at the house almost every month. The number gathered would vary from 20 to 50 guests. Any idea was a good excuse to have a gathering. Of course the main draw was the food. We made the food ourselves from scratch using magazines and cookbooks for ideas.

Eventually we put together a 3-ring binder of regularly used recipes. All the food at the party was vegetarian. There was no animal flesh.

In sixth grade, I wrote a term paper. My topic was the meaning of a vegetarian diet. I learned that "vegetarian" meant living which gave me some relief. I always thought it meant vegetables. I am sure in my youth I ate a lot of vegetables but I ate even more grains, beans and cheese. Every dinner had to have potato or rice or noodles or beans with cheese.

One of our favorite dishes was Barley Casserole. It was a combination of barley, mushrooms and broth. I would eat bowls of the casserole and have a little green salad on the side.

Barley Casserole

1 cup barley, soaked overnight with 3 inches of kombu seaweed
1 cup chopped mushrooms
½ cup carrot, peeled and chopped coarsely
½ cup celery, chopped coarsely
1 bay leaf
7 sprigs of thyme
2 cups water or vegetable broth
¾ teaspoon salt

Preheat oven to 350°F.
Reserve kombu. Rinse barley. Put barley, mushrooms, carrot, celery, kombu seaweed, bay leaf and thyme into a six-quart baking dish. Add water.

Cover and bake 45 minutes or until water is absorbed and barley is tender. Remove kombu, bay leaf and sprigs of thyme. Stir in salt. Serve warm.

Around the age of 18, I decided that if I was going to call myself a vegetarian, I was going to stop eating all animal flesh. Chicken and fish and bacon walked off my plate. However, I still ate eggs and dairy, and allowed for animal broths.

To get a better idea of being vegetarian, I studied

different diet ideologies. Some of them I tried. The first diet or

eating style I tried was restricted to plant-based foods grown

above the ground.

Sundays at our house was Pancake Day. My father was

the cook. My father's basic pancake recipe was a mixture of

grains – rye, oats, and any other grain available, freshly

ground. He would use buttermilk, vegetable water or beer,

and add in an egg.

Martin's Pancakes

1 cup flour – rye, corn, millet, barley, buckwheat, whole
wheat,   rolled oats (always in combination)
1 cup liquid - milk, vegetable water, beer
1 egg
1 teaspoon baking soda
¼ teaspoon sea salt

Spoon onto a heated cast iron or non-stick pan to desired
size. Cook over medium high heat until bubbles form on
the top and the underside is slightly brown. Turn over,
and brown on the other side. Serve warm.

With this diet I was trying, my father listened to its restrictions. He then looked at my mother; she simply encouraged him to do his best. We worked together to create a pancake within those limitations. It was flat and turned out to be tasteless cardboard. So much for plant-based pancakes!

One day, when my brother and I were alone in the house, we got hungry. Since no one was there to help us with food, we set about preparing ourselves something to eat. Since I was not sure what to do for food preparation, I turned it over to my brother.

Neither of us were the cooking type, so my brother put things together that normally did not go together. I do not remember what we ate. I only know that at the end of the meal, our bellies were full and we were content. That day I learned the concept of **creative food combining**.

Later I found out that my grandfather was a very creative cook. It may have been because he survived the

French concentration camp during World War One or living on a farm in Iowa where there was only so much food variety. My father inherited this ability and passed it down to some of his children.

I have heard the idea of trying out a new recipe before a special event but I tend to use my dinner guests as co-food-testers with me. I like company when I am trying something new.

Creative cooking required two things: the willingness to try something new and an idea of how flavors meld with each other. During her time of studying chemistry, my eldest sister made a comment that stuck with me:

"Baking is a lot like chemistry - once you know how the chemicals or ingredients combine, you can change them to create other dishes."

Surviving Japan

Just before I turned 21 years old, I was invited to study Japanese in Japan for nine months. I would live with a host family. I figured it would be easy, after all, they eat a plant-based diet with a little bit of fish, right? Wrong. Being a vegetarian almost cost me my trip. Nobody wanted to cook for a vegetarian. Most dishes Japanese made contained some type of animal, especially fish broth.

I learned that the Japanese consume animal in every meal and in most dishes – very similar to the American diet in which a salad needs to have bacon bits and vegetables soup is made from meat broth. In Japan's case, sea critters flavor most of their dishes even to the point of having dried fish shavings over tofu.

In order not to lose my opportunity, I told the school that I would cook for myself. (I figured I could wing it. How difficult could it be?!)

Shortly thereafter, I stood in the living room of my Japanese host family and was introduced to the members. We had a wonderful dinner that first night. There was rice and miso soup, along with pickles and sweet beans. I have no idea what else I ate but I loved the flavors.

I wanted to experience more. I wanted to learn home cooking and share it with my family when I returned to my home. That would be quite a return gift. I was on cloud nine. It was the first and the last meal they cooked for me.

The following morning, the host mother showed me the variety of vegetables she had in her refrigerator and the fact that she had a pot of cooked rice. Japanese eat rice, miso soup, salad and fish for a traditional breakfast or they have toast, salad and maybe a soft boiled egg for a conventional breakfast. I stood staring at the drawer of vegetables. What on earth was I going to do with the vegetables? I had to do some fast thinking.

My host mother showed me the basics of making miso soup – miso, fish broth, wakame seaweed, and a few pieces of tofu. This was not going to work for me; I would starve with type of broth. I flashed back to my mother.

I had watched my mother make vegetable soup enough times to have an idea of how I could enhance the miso soup.

Joan's Vegetable Soup

3 potatoes, washed and cut into quarters
2 stalks of celery, sliced diagonally
1 brown onion, peeled and chopped into bite size pieces
1 large can of stewed tomatoes, cut into chunks
1 bay leaf
1 teaspoon of sea salt
3 cups of water

Put in a pressure cooker. Cook under pressure for 3 minutes. Reduce pressure and open lid.

Add 3 cups of chopped green cabbage. Cover pot for 10 minutes. Reduce pressure and open lid. Serve warm.

Remove bay leaf and serve.

I was given a 1-quart sauce pan to make my soup. I packed it full of chopped vegetables, some seaweed and tofu. I added water to the level of the vegetables and cooked it until the vegetables were soft. I then added miso.

My breakfast from that day on was miso "stew" and rice. It was excellent.

Miso Stew

1 small yam, peeled and diced small
3 inches of daikon radish, peeled and diced small
Handful of young spinach, washed
1 thick slice of onion, chopped into bite size pieces
1/3 cup tofu chunks
Small amount of wakame seaweed.
Water to the level of the vegetables.

Bring to boil. Simmer until vegetables are soft. Mix 1 Tablespoon of miso in a small amount of broth. Add to stew. Serve warm.

It was a challenge for people to feed me when I was a guest at other people's homes. When I found a dish I liked, I would ask how it was made.

Japanese Potato Salad

1 boiled red potato, skin removed, chopped into bite size pieces
1 small sweet apple, peeled, core removed, chopped into bite size pieces
¼ cup carrot, peeled and chopped into small pieces
1 Tablespoon mayonnaise
Salt, to flavor

Combine all ingredients in a bowl. Serve either at room temperature or chill for 1 hour before serving. Salad is best eaten the same day.

I ate a lot of squash, kabocha, which literally means pumpkin. It was boiled and stirred with a sauce of soy sauce and sugar.

<u>Kabocha</u>

1 kabocha, deseeded, peeled and chopped into bite size chunks
1-part soy sauce and 1-part sugar to form a sauce

Put squash in a pan and cover with water. Bring to a boil. Cook until soft. Drain liquid. Mix the soy sauce and sugar together in a small bowl. Pour over squash and stir to coat. Serve warm.

Weekly Fasting

When I came home from Japan, I began fasting weekly for 24 hours. How do I handle starving on a fasting day? I enjoy lots of weak hot tea - and I cook. Probably not the thought you had, but it worked for me.

Since food was the only thing on my mind, I used this time to try different recipes. I got really exuberant. I usually made too much food so leftovers carried us through another meal or two. I cooked so much through the afternoon that by the time my fast was over and I could eat dinner, I was not hungry.

Instead of tasting the food to determine if it was spiced right, I developed my sense of smell; and I think smelling the food for hours filled me up. All the dishes I prepared were vegetarian.

I did some experimenting with weekly meal planning. I found that two days of meals would feed us for the week. I also found that ingredients were being wasted since several of the dishes on the list were never made. After attempting meal planning for six weeks, the idea was abandoned.

Other Influences - Weekly leftovers

During the first six months of studying Traditional Oriental Medicine to become an Acupuncturist, I rented a room near the school. I would return home on weekends.

At that time, I would do my laundry; and before I left, my mother would clean out the refrigerator of all leftover fruits and vegetables. These items became my food for the following week.

Soy sauce, oil and a couple of spices were all the kitchen supplies I had. I boiled. I sautéed. I ate raw. My meals were very simple in those months.

Indian Food

When I was in Japan, because of my vegetarian ways, my family and friends would take me to Indian restaurants. This was my first time eating Indian food and it was good.

When I returned home from Japan, Japanese cooking was my usual routine for months. When I got tired of Japanese food, I learned how to cook Indian food. I purchased several books: The Vegetarian Table India by Yamuna Devi, What's Cooking Indian by Shehzad Husain, and Dakshi: Vegetarian Delicacies from South India by Chandra Padmanabhan. Each book had a recipe that became a regular dish at the family dinner table.

While studying for my doctorate in Homeopathic Medicine in Santa Monica, one of the teachers talked about healing patients through a temporary change to their diet. The patient prepares a large amount dal and eats the same dal for ten days.

Dal is a legume soup made from dried peas, beans or lentils and maybe some vegetables. It is the main source of protein in the Indian diet, and is usually eaten with vegetables, rice or flatbread.

Mung Dal

½ cup mung dal split
¼ cup urid (black) dal split
3 cups stock or water
3 cups zucchini, shredded
1 brown onion, chopped
2 cloves garlic, chopped
2 cups canned stewed tomatoes, chopped
Bring to a boil in a pan. Then simmer until lentils are slightly tender.

In a frying pan, heat on low for 1 minute:
2 Tablespoons Oil
1 teaspoon ground cumin
1 teaspoon ground coriander
¼ cup green chilies
½ teaspoon turmeric

Add to lentils. Blend until smooth 2 cups of the lentils and return to pot. Stir in:
1 ¼ cups soy milk
1 cup cooked short or medium grain brown rice

Serve warm.

Macrobiotic diet

The next diet I studied was the Macrobiotic diet. It was recommended for people with serious ailments. Having its origin in Japan, its concept was mostly cooked foods: Fifty percent of your meal is from grain, about 20 percent is from beans, 25 percent is from vegetables and the last 5 percent is from fish or fruit or dairy. The food combinations were simple. Kristine Turner Americanized the diet in her book, The Self-Healing Cookbook.

One chapter discussed an approach to weight loss that I found interesting. She noted that if you are overweight, you switch the ratios of grain and vegetables. In other words, you eat 50 percent vegetables and 25 percent grains.

Anna Marie Colbin wrote another excellent Macrobiotic book called, Whole Food Meals. This book is arranged according to seasons and gives an entire meal plan for a day that included snacks and dessert.

The idea I liked in this book was that leftovers were transformed into new dishes. In other words, the food was being recycled.

I loved the food of the Macrobiotic diet. I felt nourished and grounded. My only problem on the diet was food portion. I felt like all I was doing was eating. It could have been the fact that the meal plans were set for four people instead of 1 person. Or it could have been that having a four course meal was too much for me.

Raw food diet

Then I heard of the raw food diet, and wanted to learn more. I attended classes from Chef Rachel Carr at Cru in Los Angeles. A piece of her story is how she used raw food to help a friend lose weight.

I bought several books on how to prepare raw food. My favorites were <u>Raw Food Made Easy for 1 or 2 People</u> by Jennifer Cornbleet, <u>Rainbow Green Live-Food Cuisine</u> by Gabriel Cousens, MD and <u>Rawsome</u> by Bridgette Mars. I even used this diet for my mother to support her during a major illness. We both enjoyed the flavors of the food.

One important aspect to raw food eating is to decide what you are going to eat days ahead of time to allow for the soaking and any dehydrating needed. Good thing I had some idea of meal planning.

Only this time I was very conservative on how much food we really needed. One nice aspect to the raw food diet is that once you have combined the ingredients, since there is no cooking, it is ready to eat immediately.

Another aspect to raw food is learning to heat your food using spices instead of fire. Juliano in his book, <u>The Uncook Book</u>, used this concept often. A dish made with warm spices at room temperature can be just as comforting as

one made in the oven.

Chapter Two
Approach to Food

The crowning glory to all the years of diet study was completing a program in Chinese Nutrition from Mao Ni and Cathy McNease.

Chinese Nutrition follows the basic premise of Chinese Medicine – energy moves the body. A poorly functioning body can be greatly improved by changing the flow of the energy in the tissues and organs. And this is done through the foods we eat.

Chinese Nutrition is the use of plants and animals to support and adjust the levels of energy flowing through the channels in your body to the various organ systems. Plant and animal parts affect the function of your body. Each food can stimulate or decrease a particular function of an organ.

Understanding how food contributes to your body will help you create a depth to your eating. You will be able to apply basic healing principles at each meal to enhance and support your level of wellness. The simple approach to food is to look at its color, its flavor and the degree of warmth or coolness it creates in you when you eat it.

Color

The color of each food gives you an idea of the area it will affect in the body. Every color corresponds to an organ system, and also relates to a sense organ and to a tissue.

- Green – Liver and Gallbladder organ systems, eyes and tendons
- Red – Heart and Small Intestine organ systems, tongue and blood vessels
- Yellow – Spleen and Stomach organ systems, mouth and muscles
- White – Lung and Large Intestine organ systems, nose, skin and surface hair

- Black – Kidneys and Urinary Bladder organ systems, ear and bone

By choosing your foods according to color, you can specifically help one aspect of your body to enhance healing. If you want a general effect on the body, choose a meal that contains all the colors.

<u>Barbecue Vegetables</u>

Container #1:
½ cup mushroom, thickly sliced
½ cup crook neck squash, ¼ inch slices
½ red bell pepper, 1 1/2 inch pieces

Container #2:
½ cup asparagus, 2 inch pieces
½ cup sugar peas

In each container, add:
1 Tablespoon oregano, dried
1 Tablespoon Italian seasoning
1 Tablespoon lemon or lime juice
1 Tablespoon olive oil
¼ teaspoon salt

Prepare vegetables and let sit for 2 hours to overnight. Drain juice. Barbecue container #1 until half way cooked. Add container #2 and finish cooking. Serve warm.

If your emotions or attitude needs some help, color will also affect your mood.

- Green – soothes irritability, pent up anger and emotions
- Red – calms down over-excitement or mania but also lifts you into a joyful mood
- Yellow – soothes worry and anxiety, decreases over-thinking
- White – raises you out of grief and melancholy
- Black – quells fear and fright

Flavor

There are five flavors:

1. Bitter
2. Sweet
3. Sour
4. Salty
5. Pungent

Each flavor has an effect on an organ system, sense organ and a tissue.

- Sour – Liver and Gallbladder organ systems, eyes and tendons
- Bitter – Heart and Small Intestine organ systems, tongue and blood vessels
- Sweet – Spleen and Stomach organ systems, mouth and muscles
- Pungent – Lung and Large Intestine organ systems, nose, skin and surface hair
- Salty – Kidneys and Urinary Bladder organ systems, ear and bone

When preparing a meal, you can choose one flavor to predominate or you can use a little of each flavor to give a little support for the entire body.

Rosemary Flat Bread

½ cup almond meal
½ cup arrowroot starch
1 cup chickpea flour
½ teaspoon baking soda
¼ teaspoon salt
2 teaspoons Cream of Tartar
Mix ingredients in a bowl.

1 cup water
2 Tablespoons lemon juice
2 Tablespoons olive oil
1 Tablespoon fresh rosemary, finely chopped

Blend the liquids together. Mix in with the dry ingredients. Cook over medium high heat, turning when bottom is slightly brown. If flat bread is not completely cooked, place in a 300°F oven for 10 minutes or until the inside is fully cooked. Serve warm.

In the Flat Bread recipe above, the breakdown of flavors is as follows.

- Pungent – rosemary

- Sweet – almond, chickpea

- Salty – salt

- Sour – lemon

Bitter

Bitter dries dampness and transforms fluids; and has a cooling effect. Typical vegetables are the bitter greens.

Bok Choy	Collard greens	Dandelion greens	Mustard greens
Celery	Wild cucumber	Radish leaves	

One way of preparing these foods is to chop them up and add them to a soup.

Cooked Greens

1 cup greens, chard/collard/mixed, washed

In a large sauce pan, bring 1 quart of water to boil. Turn off heat. Add greens. Cover. Let sit for 2 -4 minutes until greens are bright green and soft. Drain. Serve warm with olive oil and salt.

Sweet/Bland

Sweet flavors harmonize and calm; and help to reduce pain. Sugar and sweet are two different creatures. Sugar can be found as a strand of molecules. Sweet is the impression the brain gets from the taste buds.

Do you have sugar issues? Is your life wrapped around every bite of food needing to be sweet? If so, it is time to get off of sugar. <u>The Perricone Prescription</u> by Nicholas Perricone, MD describes how an imbalance in blood sugar will cripple your immune system. Some form of sugar is found in all processed foods.

To get off sugar, you need to stop eating all foods made with sugar, fruit and grain products for at least 30 consecutive days.

Just because you get off sugar does not mean you remove sweet from your diet. In order to survive removing sugar from your diet you need to consume two things: sweet and fat.

Since sweet is vital to health and healing, finding sweet without sugar is the key to healthy eating. Making the most of the natural sugar found in a vegetable related to how you prepare the vegetable.

Baking your vegetables brings out the sugar and therefore, tastes the sweetest of all cooking methods. Beets, carrots, parsnips, and butternut squash are their most sweet when baked.

Baked Beets

1 beet, stems removed and washed

Heat oven to 350°F. Put beet in a baking dish and cover.
Cook for 20 to 40 minutes, until tender. Use a fork to ensure beet is cooked to the core. Remove the skin.
Serve warm or at room temperature.

Colored bell peppers and sugar snap peas also add sweetness. These are best cooked or raw. Baking does not heighten their sweetness.

When you have succeeded removing sugar from your diet, you will find the sweetness in foods you previously considered not very sweet. You may even find that baked vegetables are too sweet. One way to enjoy vegetables is by boiling them.

Boiled Carrots

1 carrot, peeled, quartered, cut into ½ inch pieces

In a small sauce pan, bring water to a boil. Add carrots. Cook for 2-4 minutes on high heat until carrots are tender. Drain. Serve warm or room temperature.

Salty

Salty flavors help to soften and reduce hardness, as well as lubricate the intestines. Obtaining a salty flavor is best achieved through sodium and potassium-rich foods. You can see that some of the foods that benefit sodium levels also benefit potassium.

A balance of sodium and potassium allows a proper amount of fluid into and between the cells and supports the bones, muscles and nervous systems. Using these foods to flavor your food may reduce your desire for too much extra salt.

Sodium-rich foods include:

Apples	Apricots – dried	Asparagus	Beets
Beet Greens	Cabbage –red	Carrots	Celery
Dandelion greens	Dulse seaweed	Horseradish	Kale
Kombu – Kelp seaweed	Lentils	Okra	Olives – black
Parsley	Sesame seeds roasted	Sunflower seeds	

Potassium-rich foods:

Almonds	Apples	Apple cider vinegar – raw	Apricots
Arugula	Bananas	Beets	Beet tops
Black Cherries	Broccoli	Blue Berries	Carrots
Cashews – raw	Cucumbers	Kale	Kombu – Kelp seaweed
Parsley	Sesame Seeds roasted	Soybeans	Swiss Chard
Tomatoes	Walnuts	Watercress	

But when you still need some salt for flavoring, add natural salt. Some common natural salts are Sea Salt, Celtic Salt, and Himalayan Salt. Not only do these salts add sodium, but they also add other minerals that will round out the flavor of your dish.

Avoid table salt when possible. Table salt has a high amount of sodium per volume without the benefit of supporting minerals. It also contains sugar to give the sodium some appeal.

I used to make this morning hot cereal:

Morning Cereal

1/3 cup Mixed 7 Grains (rice, barley, sorghum, millet)
3 inches kombu seaweed
1 ½ cups water

Combine all in a sauce pan and soak overnight. In the morning, bring to a boil and simmer 40 minutes until done. Discard seaweed. Serve warm with Earth Balance or butter.

One morning my cereal tasted bland. I added salt but it only made it taste salty. Something was missing. I realized I forgot to put the kombu seaweed in during the cooking process. To add a subtle salty flavor before I add salt, I use kombu seaweed any time I cook with liquids – vegetables, beans, and rice. I also use celery in cooked or raw dishes.

Sour

Sour foods absorb and consolidate fluid in situations where the body is being depleted by leaking fluids.

Sour foods are lemon, lime, tamarind, vinegars, umeboshi plum, sauerkraut, and dill pickles. Sour helps the stomach to digest. It also increases the amount of acid in the stomach which helps the digestive enzymes break down food.

Just adding lemon or vinegar to a dish helps to make it more digestible.

Coleslaw with Peanut Dressing

Mix together in a small bowl:
1/3 cup peanut butter
¼ cup cider vinegar
3 Tablespoons honey or agave nectar
1 ½ Tablespoons soy sauce
1 teaspoon sesame oil
1/8 teaspoon ginger powder

In a large bowl add:
5 cups green cabbage, shredded
½ cup carrot, peeled, grated
½ cup cilantro

Stir in peanut sauce. Let sit for 1 hour before serving.

Cucumber Salad

Place in a bowl. Leave in the refrigerator overnight, then drain and rinse.
1 cucumber, peeled, thinly sliced
½ teaspoon salt
Enough water to cover the cucumbers

In a bowl, mix together
Cucumber
½ teaspoon salt
2 Tablespoons red wine vinegar
1 teaspoon agave nectar
Black pepper to taste

Serve chilled or at room temperature.

Pungent

Pungent foods help to smooth and facilitate circulation.

They open the pores of the skin and allow sweating to take

place, especially in times of common cold or flu.

Pungent foods are chili peppers, onion, garlic,

asparagus and such spices as ginger, wasabi, peppermint,

caraway and black pepper.

A little addition of pungent flavor helps circulation and induces sweating.

Caraway Cabbage

1 carrot, peeled, diagonally sliced
1 stalk celery, diced into ½ inch pieces
1 ½ cup cabbage, cut in 1 ½ inch pieces
½ teaspoon caraway seeds
1 Tablespoon olive oil

Heat wok over medium high heat. Add carrots and ½ cup of water. Cover and cook for 4 minutes or until barely tender. Uncover wok. Add celery and cabbage. Cook for 3 minutes, stirring as needed. Add caraway seeds. Stir for 2 minutes. Remove wok from heat. Stir in olive oil and salt to taste. Serve warm.

Temperature

Temperature is the effect the food has during its digestion. Fruits are the coldest. Vegetables tend to be cooling. Beans, nuts and seeds tend to be neutral to warm. Along with the natural temperature, you can add heat to a food through the cooking process. Cooking fruit, changes it from cold to cool. Lightly steaming your food will increase

heat less than if you baked the item.

You might have already noticed that your body gives

you hints on the temperature of the food it desires. In

summer, you could be craving salads; in winter you may want

soups. If you have a cold, you may desire spicy foods; this is

one way the body heats itself up to push the cold out through

your pores.

Below is a chart of the temperature of selected

vegetables in their raw form.

Cold	Cool	Neutral	Warm
Chinese Cabbage	Artichoke	Chard	Bell Pepper
Mung Bean Sprouts	Asparagus	Lettuce	Green Beans
Sea Weed	Broccoli	Shitake Mushroom	Kale
Snow Pea	All types of squash	Sweet Potato	Parsley
White mushroom	Turnip	Yam	Garlic (Hot)

Balanced Meal

I always consider color, flavor, and overall degree of heat I want to experience for my meal. I like my plate to be colorful.

But depending on my need of the day or available food, it might be monochrome – a white, an orange, a green.

Additionally, I consider where and how long a food is grown.

In putting a dish together, I collect as many items to fit these descriptions as possible.

- Grown under the ground
- Grown on a vine
- Growing cycle requires months to mature
- Growing cycle matures in weeks
- Item is leafy
- Item is dense
- Item is grown in water

Both ways are good. Just know what you are eating. I

tend to use a variety of color to add more nutrients.

Occasionally, I do monochrome of either orange or green.

A green and white dish could be composed of noodles,

grilled asparagus, green beans and broccoli that was cooked in

a kelp broth and drained, with tahini drizzled over the top

and a sprinkling of salt and pepper.

Today's Lunch

1 zucchini, bite size pieces
1 crook neck squash, bite sized pieces
1 carrot, peeled, diced
3 small stalks of celery, diagonally sliced
3 mushrooms, chopped small
½ cup butternut squash, peeled, bite size pieces
1 bok choy, baby size
3 Tablespoons split mung bean lentils
3 inches kombu seaweed
1 bay leaf
2 cups water

Add to pressure cooker. Cook in pressure cooker
for 3 minutes. Reduce pressure and open lid.
Discard seaweed and bay leaf.
Add as desired: salt, olive oil. Serve warm.

How does the above recipe fit my meal qualifications?

- Something grown under the ground – carrot
- Something grown on a vine – butternut squash, zucchini, crook neck squash, mung bean
- Something that takes months to grow – butternut squash, mung bean
- Something that matures in weeks – bok choy, zucchini, crook neck squash, mushroom, celery
- Something that is leafy – bok choy, seaweed, bay leaf
- Something that is dense – butternut squash, mung bean
- Something grown in water – seaweed

Whether I use one dish or several, I use this same theory in building all my meals.

Chapter Three
Building a Dish

A man, who was overweight and had allergies, wanted help with his diet. I recommended that he temporarily stop eating the nightshade family – potatoes, tomatoes, eggplant, bell peppers; and stop eating any corn products. His response was, "Then what is there to eat?"

His concern was not about the potatoes but about the corn. His regular diet consisted of corn tortillas, beans and meat. He had eaten this way for so many years that he did not consider other foods.

It is easy to enter the grocery store or go straight to your usual aisles. It also can be daunting to look in the produce aisles. All the fruits and vegetables are laid out to create a beautiful display. Some produce is bunched together because it is usually cooked together, like some of your stir fry ingredients – bean sprouts, ginger, bamboo shoots and water chestnuts.

Sometimes the produce people have ideas on how to prepare the different vegetables but that can be rare. The first step to increasing your list of edible produce is to have a name of a vegetable. Sometimes a list helps one to realize there are other vegetables available besides potatoes and corn.

I handed him this chart:

VEGETABLES			
Alfalfa Sprout	Carrot	Kohlrabi	Romaine Lettuce
Artichoke	Cauliflower	Lettuce	Seaweed – Nori, Dulse, Kombu
Asparagus	Celery	Lotus Root	Snow Pea/Snap Pea
Avocado	Chard	Luffa Squash	Soybean Sprout
Bamboo Shoots	Napa Cabbage	Mushroom - Button	Spinach
Barley Sprouts	Cilantro	Mushroom - Ganoderma	Sweet Potato/Yam
Beet/Beet Greens	Corn	Mushroom - Shitake	Taro
Bell Pepper	Cucumber	Mushroom - White	Turnip/Turnip Greens
Bitter Greens	Radish	Mustard Greens	Water Chestnut
Bitter Melon	Dandelion	Olive	Watercress
Black Fungus - Wood Ears	Eggplant	Parsley	White Fungus - Silver Ears
Bok Choy	Fennel Root	Parsnip	Winter Melon
Broccoli	Leafy Greens	Potato	Zucchini/Summer Squash
Brussel Sprout	Green Bean/ String Bean	Pumpkin/ Winter Squash	
Burdock Root	Jicama	Radish	
Cabbage	Kale	Rice Sprouts	
BEANS			
All kinds of Beans	Garbanzo	Lima	Soybean/Tofu
Azuki (Red)	Kidney	Mung	
Black	Lentil	Pea	
NUTS & SEEDS			
Almond	Flax Seed	Pine Nut	Sunflower Seed
Black Sesame Seed	Kernel	Pistachio	Walnut
Chestnut	Lotus Seed	Pumpkin Seed	Winter Melon Seed
Filbert	Peach	Sesame Seed	

The chart helped him to see that there is a variety of food available to eat that may be what he is already eating.

The only difference is that now the special item that is saved for rare occasions may become the daily dish.

My mother regularly talked about the turnips and mashed rutabaga she ate in her youth. Until I looked into alternatives for white potatoes, they never found their way to my dining table. Now, I add them in rotation to the other root vegetables.

The chart above shows you a variety of food options for vegetables, beans, nuts and seeds. Your percent of each category can be roughly:

- 50-75% or 3 cups of vegetables
- 15-25% or ¼ cup - 1 cup of beans
- 10% or 1 – 4 tablespoons of nuts and seeds
- 5-10% or ¼ - ½ cup of "other" animal products, grain, fruit

You can follow this guideline per day or per meal.

Considerations in creating a dish

When you think about food, do you want it raw or

cooked?

Raw?
>A salad?
>A smoothie?
>Vegetables and dip?

Cooked?
>Steamed?
>Stir fried?
>Boiled?
>Baked?

Now look at the food you have on hand, or create a list

and go shopping. Start with the vegetables.

How do you want your vegetables?

>On the side?
>As the main attraction?
>On top?
>Underneath?

Next, think about beans. Is this a bean day?

>Will you make them a side dish?
>Do you want to use as a bed to hold the vegetables?

Shall you include them in the cooking of the vegetables?

What about nuts and seeds? How will you have them?

As a little crunch?
As a lot of flavor?
As a cream sauce?
For dessert?

Now to finish the dish, if you did not add any nuts,

seeds or avocado, you may want to add a little oil.

Food without any fat will not be satisfying. Fat gives

you a feeling of satisfaction and satiation after a meal. Without

fat, you may start looking for sugar to fill the void. When you

eat fat with your meals, you crave less sweet.

A little fat goes a long way but each person's idea of

little is different. Add the amount you want.

When I ate meals in Greece, my plate would always

come with the vegetables sitting in 3 tablespoons of olive oil.

If you are having problems with what food goes together, imitate what you know. Looking at various cuisines may also help you to determine combinations.

Below are popular ingredients found in various cuisines. You may notice that there are some redundancies in ingredients.

- **American**
  - Peas, carrots, potatoes, broccoli, corn, dried beans
- **German**
  - Potatoes, cabbage
- **Hungarian**
  - Cabbage, potato, cucumber, green beans
- **Indian**
  - Cauliflower, eggplant, green peas, cabbage, potato, spinach, rice, dried peas and lentils
- **Italian**
  - Pasta, tomatoes, zucchini, eggplant, bell pepper
- **Japanese and Chinese**
  - Mushroom, mung bean sprouts, snow pea, bok choy, cucumber, kabocha
- **Mexican**
  - Avocado, lime, corn, rice, dried beans

To expand your list of possible food items, start with the foods you know. You may already have ideas on how to prepare them. Then on a weekly basis buy a different item to incorporate.

If you use potatoes, substitute a turnip or rutabaga the next time you make the dish. If you normally use black beans, try using garbanzo beans. If you usually use almonds, what will pistachios or pine nuts do for the dish?

This substitution method will allow you to taste the versatility in your dish using other ingredients or inspire you on to create a brand new dish all together.

Portion size

The same food can get boring. Keep your portions to a trial size. This will allow you to taste it and have it for one or two meals.

By doing this, you will know whether the dish needs to be eaten right away or whether it is better made the day ahead.

Keeping notes

If you make a dish for the next day, write down what ingredients you used, how much, and how did you prepare it. Simple notes will allow you to make adjustments as needed or remind you how made the dish so you can duplicate it exactly.

Chapter Four
Spicing it Up

Now that you have ideas of what major ingredients to put in a dish, the next part is how to spice them, or not spice them at all. The American diet is filled with recipes that have butter, salt and pepper. Or translated: oil, salt and pepper.

If you already run hot, you may choose to leave out the pepper. If there is enough fat in the dish by way of avocado or nuts, you may skip the oil. If you want a simple and subtle taste, you may omit the salt as well. Spice your food according to your body's need at the moment.

Viewing the spice section in the grocery store is both exciting and overwhelming. The variety is amazing and the uses are endless.

Cookbooks will use multiple spices in a given recipe; and recommend various spices to keep on hand.

Spices are a food. Even though they are dried, they are good for only so long. My rule of thumb is if they have no smell, the spice has lost its flavor and is too old to use. Or on occasion, the spice smells rancid. I donate those spices to the compost pile.

Some spices are best packaged like cinnamon, cumin and turmeric.

Other spices are best fresh – bay leaf, oregano, thyme, and rosemary.

For those herbs that are seasonal – basil, dill and cilantro, you can grow them fresh during the summer and use them in their dried state during the rest of the year.

Ground or Whole

Ground versions of herbs like cumin and nutmeg will lose their quality faster than the seed version. Having the seeds on hand with a spice grinder, will allow you versatility in which you can use them ground or whole.

When you want the flavor to permeate the entire dish, use the ground form. When you want occasional bites of more intense flavor, use the whole form.

Raw or Cooked

Herbs react differently depending on whether they are cooked or raw. Raw dishes require more herbs, as much as a tablespoon, to add flavoring; while cooked dishes need only a teaspoon of the same herb to impart its flavor.

Fresh Herbs

When I use fresh herbs in cooking, I use the entire branch. I clean it well and lay the branches on top of the food I am cooking or in the cooking water. When the dish is ready, I discard the herb, stem and all. If a few leaves have separated from the stem, I leave them in the dish.

Getting to know herbs and spices

One way of getting to know herbs is to limit a dish to one herb or spice. This will help you to a have clearer understanding of the effect the herb has on food.

Start with a spice with which you are familiar. Try it with cooked a vegetable dish; in a salad; and with a pot of beans. By tasting it prepared different ways, you will discover how you prefer to use this spice. You will also find out how much you need.

Build your stash of spices one at a time. A cupboard of many spices is not better than a trusted few. As you acquire the spices you like, use them in combination with each other.

Below is a list of spices used in various cuisines. By using these spices, you add an ethnic flair to your choice of ingredients.

- **American**
    - Oregano, dill, sage, rosemary, parsley, bay leaf, cinnamon
- **German**
    - Caraway seeds
- **Hungarian**
    - Paprika
- **Indian**
    - Ginger, cardamom, curry, cumin, turmeric, cinnamon
- **Italian**
    - Basil, oregano, olive oil
- **Japanese and Chinese**
    - Ginger, sesame, soy sauce
- **Mexican**
    - Cumin, cilantro, chilies

Cooked Cabbage

1 cup green cabbage, finely sliced
½ cup carrots, grated
¼ celery, thinly sliced
½ teaspoon caraway seeds
2 teaspoons olive oil
Salt and pepper as desired

Sauté cabbage over medium high heat in a non-stick pan for 1 minute. Add carrots, celery, and caraway seeds. Stir until cabbage is wilted. Remove from heat. Stir in olive oil, salt and pepper. Serve warm.

Hungarian Vegetables

1 small potato, cleaned, cut into ½ inch pieces
¼ cup bell pepper, cut into ½ inch pieces
½ cup zucchini, ¼ inch half rounds
1 cup cabbage, thinly sliced
3-inch kombu seaweed
1 teaspoon paprika
½ cup water

Put above ingredients in a pressure cooker and cook for 2 minutes. Reduce pressure and remove lid. Add
¼ teaspoon salt
1 tablespoon olive oil

Serve warm.

Chapter Five
Kitchen Tools

Your kitchen can be as elaborate or as simple as you want it to be. Start with the tools and equipment to make the food that you like.

What are your favorite foods? How are they prepared? Look at some recipes of the foods you like and see what kind of kitchen gadgets and pans are required. Occasionally these items come with suggested use or recipes. See if you like any of them and add them to your collection of possible dishes to make.

Other types of tools you may want are the ones that will make the job easier. When I say easier, it could mean less physically tasking or less time consuming, or both. This could be an assortment of cutting blades or nonstick pads for the bottom of pans or small appliances that you can preprogram to operate at a later time.

The important concept to making food is to enjoy the process. If you enjoy what you are doing, you are more apt to continue doing it.

Knives

One of our basic meals growing up was coleslaw and baked potatoes. This required chopping up the green cabbage. Our set of knives contained an 11-inch chief's knife. That was quite a feat to master but I managed to do all sorts of tasks using this rather long knife.

Martin's Coleslaw

1/3 cup sour cream
2/3 cup mayonnaise
¼ cup apple cider vinegar
1 teaspoon Dijon mustard
½ teaspoon sea salt
2 teaspoons honey

Mix in a small bowl until smooth. Set aside.

½ head of a small green cabbage, finely chopped
¼ cup brown onion, finely chopped (optional)
1 carrot, shredded (optional)

Put vegetables in a large bowl. Add the sour cream sauce
and toss until cabbage is coated.
If you want your cabbage to be soft, let stand for 1 hour
before serving. Serve chilled or at room temperature.

I use two knives for most of my food preparation:

- 8-inch chef knife
- Paring knife

I keep my knives sharp by using a hand sharpener. Electric ones are available also. Once you learn the technique of sharpening, whether by hand or by machine, it is wise to sharpen your blades before using them. If you make a habit of doing this, you will only spend about 30 seconds sharpening.

A dull knife compels you to put pressure in directions that might cause the knife to slip and cut your hand/fingers. You want your knife to move easily through the food you are cutting. You want the blade to do most of the work, not your arm muscle.

Wooden and plastic utensils

Start your collection with a **large spoon**, a **flat paddle** for pushing food around while stir frying, and a **ladle**. You may need more than one of these if you prepare more than one dish at a time.

Other equipment

A **food processor** is nice when you have limited time or your ability to cut certain thinness and styles is beyond your skill or desire. This was the lifesaver for me. I could make a chopped salad in 15 minutes, from washing the vegetables to the clean-up.

<u>Chopped Salad</u>

1 celery stalk, julienne slice
1 carrot, peeled, medium grate
1 red bell pepper, thinly sliced
1 parsnip, peeled, finely grated
1 golden beet, peeled, finely grated

Toss together with oil, vinegar, salt and pepper or your favorite salad dressing.

Best prepared an hour before eating. Serve chilled or at room temperature

---

When my hands were riddled with pain, I got very creative with the food processor. I simplified my food cleaning techniques; and I put to use all the standard blades and specialty blades that came with the food processer - chopping, slicing, julienne slicing, and grating.

The cut of the vegetable verses the flavor

It was a great time to experiment with the cut of the vegetable and how it tastes. Food has a different flavor depending on the way you cut it.

For example, think about an almond. How does it taste whole; chopped up into small pieces; ground into flour; or made into nut butter? Each one has a different flavor and is used for a different purpose. Knowing this, you can make many dishes that taste different using the same ingredients.

Get the size food processor that works for you. I use a Cuisinart food processor and have for years. My current one has a six cup capacity.

A **pressure cooker** is a pot that cooks food under pressure. This allows your food to be ready in a shorter amount of time, keeping more nutrients in the food than if you boiled it in a regular pan.

There are aluminum pressure cookers and stainless steel pressure cookers. Since aluminum has been linked to brain/ mental issues, I recommend the stainless steel.

Pressure cookers come in different sizes. I have an 8-quart pan. It seems big for one or two people but the roominess of it allows me to make large pots of soup or apple sauce if I get too exuberant with the amount of ingredients; but it also allows me to cook a half cup of beans.

Pumpkin Bean Stew

½ cup of dried mixed beans, soak overnight with a 3-inch piece of kombu, drain (save the seaweed) and rinse beans repeatedly until the water has no bubbles
1 cup butternut squash, peeled and cut into chunks
1 cup mushrooms, chopped
¾ cup water
4 sprigs rosemary

Layer into your pressure cooker, water, beans, squash and mushrooms. Lay the seaweed and rosemary on top. Cook according to pressure cooker guidelines. Release pressure and open lid. Discard rosemary and seaweed. Add ¼ teaspoon of salt or to taste. Serve warm.

A **wok** is a good pan for stir frying and sautéing. The shape of the wok allows the heat to be transferred to the sides of the pan creating more cooking area. I use an 11-inch non-stick pan. This pan is versatile for cooking for one or a crowd of eight. When cooking vegetables, they cook down in volume. The larger size pan allows you to stir a large volume of food without it falling over the edge.

Asparagus Stir Fry

½ pound asparagus, washed, snap off woody ends
1 teaspoon olive oil
Salt as desired

Heat the wok on medium high heat. When the wok is hot, add the asparagus. Stir occasionally for 2 minutes. Cover wok.
Reduce heat to low and cook for 1 minute.
When cooked, remove wok from heat.
Add oil and salt. Serve warm.

A 6-quart or larger pot is good for boiling water. It

works for making pasta, as well as boiling or steaming

vegetables.

Korean Yam Noodles or Bean Thread Noodles

Bring water to boil. Add 1 – 2 ounces of noodles. Remove pan from heat. Let stand for 10 minutes. Drain water.
Serve warm with oil and salt or added to a vegetable dish.
Serve cold with a dressing and or vegetable medley.

To vary the flavor of the noodles, use leftover cooking water from steamed or boiled vegetables.

Serve warm or at room temperature.

A **rice cooker** is versatile. Not only can you cook rice but you can cook other grains too. You can also make a rice/legume combination.

<u>Rice with Lentils</u>

1/3 cup brown short grain rice
1/3 cup white colored split peas and/or lentils
3-inch piece of kelp/Kombu
1-inch ginger root, peeled and finely grated
½ teaspoon turmeric
1 bay leaf
3 cups water

Soak rice, peas/lentils and seaweed overnight. Drain and rinse. Reserve the seaweed. Add rice/bean mixture to rice cooker. Add water, ginger, turmeric and bay leaf. Top with seaweed. Cook as directed. Discard seaweed and bay leaf.
Serve warm.

A **blender** is good for making shakes and smoothies, pureeing soups, making almond flour and making nut butters. I use the Vitamix blender.

Fruit Smoothie

8-12-ounces almond milk, depending on desired thickness
1 banana
½ apple
½ cup berries
1 ½ Tablespoons hemp protein powder
1 ½ teaspoons coconut butter
1 ½ Tablespoons almond butter

Put all ingredients into a blender. Blend until smooth. Serve immediately.

A **food dehydrator** may seem like an oddity but with my history of eating raw food, I still make some of the recipes.

I regularly buy raw nuts in bulk. I use the dehydrator as a way of preserving their freshness. I soak the nuts overnight in water. Then rinse and dehydrate. This gives the nuts a crunchy flavor. Nuts are great for snacking or adding to salads or cooked food.

Tomato Crackers

9 ounces raw almonds, soak overnight and rinse
4.5 ounces raw pumpkin seeds, soak overnight and rinse
2 ounces dried tomatoes, soak for 2 hours, reserve liquid
½ teaspoon salt
Water, as needed

In a food processor, add nuts, seeds, tomatoes, and salt. Process until smooth.
Add tomato water and plain water for a thick but spreadable consistency.

Spread on Teflon sheets to a thickness of ¼ inch.
Score into desired cracker size.
Dehydrate for 2 hours on 145°F, then reduce to 115°F.
Turn crackers over and put on screens when the top is dry, about 4 hours. Total drying time about 8 hours. Store in airtight container.

A **sieve** is handy for removing peels and other chunky items after you have cooked the food. When I make apple sauce, I remove the core, cut the apples into chunks, and pressure cook the apples. After cooking, I use the sieve to remove the peels and smooth out any lumps.

Creamy Rutabaga

3 large rutabagas, peeled and cut into chunks
Olive oil
Salt

In a sauce pan, heat water to a boil. Add rutabagas. Reduce to low heat. Cook until rutabagas are soft, about 7 minutes. Drain. Put through the sieve using the smallest whole size blade. Mix rutabaga with a small amount of olive oil and salt. Serve warm.

Apple Sauce

1 pound sweet apples, washed and cut into quarters
3 inches of kombu seaweed
½ cup water

Add apples, seaweed and water to the pressure cooker and cook under pressure for 3 minutes. Release pressure. Remove kombu. Strain apples from liquid and put into a sieve. Sieve out skins and seeds. Serve warm or at room temperature.

Chapter Six
Incorporating Beans

My favorite dinner after a swim workout when I was young was refried beans with a large portion of cheese on top. Accompanied with an iceberg salad, it was the perfect meal.

Refried Beans

1 ½ cups dried kidney beans, soaked overnight
1 onion, chopped
1 small can stewed tomatoes
1 clove garlic, minced
1 teaspoon chili powder
Pinch of cayenne pepper
5 cups water or stock
1 teaspoon salt

Put in a crock pot: kidney beans, ½ cup onion, ¼ cup tomatoes, ½ garlic minced, chili powder, cayenne pepper and 5 cups of water. Cook until beans are tender.

In a frying pan, sauté remaining onion and garlic until transparent. Add remaining tomatoes and cook for 3 minutes. Mash beans with a fork and add to frying pan. Add salt to taste. Cover and cook for 10 minutes. Serve warm.

Refried Beans – Pressure Cooked

1 sprig fresh oregano
1 cup pinto beans, soaked overnight and drained
3 inches Kombu seaweed
8 ounces of chopped tomatoes
1 cup water

Add above ingredients to pressure cooker. Cook under pressure for 6 minutes. Release pressure and open lid. Use a slotted spoon to scoop out beans. Mash beans in batches on a plate using a fork. Transfer beans to a heated skillet. Add salt to taste. Heat beans using the bean water to keep beans mixture from getting too thick. Serve warm.

One year, my grandmother came to visit with us for a few weeks. On one of those days it happened to rain. We rode our bikes home from school in the rain and were sopping wet. She greeted us at the back door with towels and a cup of hot chocolate she made from scratch. When we had gotten out of our wet school clothes, she gave us bowls of split pea soup.

Split Pea Soup

In a large soup pan, put in:
8 cups water
2 cups split green peas, washed
1 stalk celery, chopped
1 large carrot, ¼ inch pieces
½ teaspoon thyme, ground
A pinch of cayenne pepper and 1 bay leaf

Bring to a boil. Boil for 20 minutes. Lower heat to sim. Continue cooking until peas are tender. Add salt and pepper to taste. Serve warm.

The Legume Family

Beans, peas and lentils make up the legume family.

- When I think of beans, I think of a side of beans, bean soup and burritos.
- When I think of peas, I think of soup.
- When I think of lentils, I think of a side of lentils or a soup.

Legumes can be eaten individually or in combination. Mixed beans give a medley of different flavors with each bite.

Most large grocery chains have a typical array of legumes: black beans, lima beans, kidney beans, navy beans, mixed beans, Pinto beans, green peas and brown Lentils.

But when you go to ethnic grocery stores, Mexican, Korean, Japanese, Indian, you are exposed to other varieties. This is where the fun begins.

Basil Moong Soup

Soak for 8 hours:
2/3 cup moong lentils
3 inches of kombu seaweed
Water for soaking

Reserve seaweed. Rinse and drain lentils until there are no bubbles in the rinse water. Add to pressure cooker:
Soaked lentils
Reserved kombu
1 ½ cups of water
¼ cup basil leaves, fresh

Cook under pressure for 5 minutes. Release pressure and open lid. Remove seaweed. Add salt as desired. Serve warm.

Green & Black Beans

Soak for 8 hours:
½ cup black beans
3 inches kombu seaweed
Soaking water

Reserve seaweed. Rinse beans. Add to pressure cooker:
Soaked beans
Reserved seaweed

Cook under pressure for 11 minutes. Release pressure and open lid. Add to pot:
1 cup green beans, cut into 1 ½ inch pieces
1 small carrot, peeled, cut into ½ pieces
1 stalk celery, diced ½ inch pieces
1 cup green cabbage, cut into 1 inch chunks
3 mushroom, sliced
Large handful, oregano sprigs

Cook under pressure for 2 minutes. Release pressure and open lid. Remove seaweed. Stir in ½ teaspoon salt. Serve warm.

Soaking

The most popular reason for not eating beans is because they cause intestinal bloating and gas for a large portion of the population.

If you are one of those people, soaking your beans before using them will cut down on the bloating and gas. Soaking is recommended for the larger legumes, but I use it for all beans, peas and legumes – the whole family. The soaking process I use is a combination of two methods:

I soak the legumes overnight in fresh water with a 3-inch piece of kombu seaweed added. When the legumes have finished soaking, I save the seaweed.

I drain the beans and put them into a large pan. I then add water slowly to the pan stirring the beans around with my hand. I continue this until the water fills the bowl. I drain the water and begin the process again until there are little to no bubbles that appear during the rinsing cycle. Getting rid of the bubbles reduces the gas factor. Garbanzo beans and lentils create a large amount of bubbles.

One of the reasons for not soaking the smaller legumes is that they easily sprout. The raw food diet recommends sprouting beans to unleash their vitality and make them more digestible.

You can purposely sprout a bean by soaking it for 8 hours, then changing the water and soaking it through the next day.

I have unintentionally sprouted beans because of a change of schedule. To keep the beans fresh, I put them in the refrigerator with a change of water.

Sometime I have changed the water for 2 days before I was able to use the beans. If the beans are whole, they usually have sprouted. The small sprout does not change the flavor of the legume. I cook the beans as I had intended.

Mixed Lentils

2/3 cup mixed lentils and split peas, soaked overnight
3-inch piece kombu seaweed
1 bay leaf
3 cups water
1 Tablespoon olive oil
Salt

Bring to a boil: water, lentils mixture, kombu, and bay leaf. Simmer until tender. Discard bay leaf and kombu. Add olive oil and salt as desired. Serve warm.

Red Lentils

Soak for 8 hours:
2/3 cups red lentils
3 inches kombu seaweed
Soaking water

Reserve seaweed. Rinse and drain lentils. Add to pressure cooker:
Soaked lentils
Reserved kombu
1 1/3 cup water

Cook under pressure for 2 minutes. Reduce pressure and open lid. Discard kombu. Add salt as desired. Serve warm.

Legumes can be used by themselves or added to other dishes. They are good as a side dish, as the bed to lay vegetables on, or in place of bread.

If you find that your beans are sticking to the bottom of the pressure cooker but you do not need more water, cook the beans under pressure for half the amount of time. Then turn off the burner and let the pressure cooker depressurize on its own. It will take about 5 minutes. During this slow depressurization, the beans are still cooking but without the intense heat from the burner.

Another way of using beans is when they are ground into flour. You can substitute a small portion of the flour in a recipe for bean flour or you can find recipes that use only bean flour, such as the Indian flat bread called 'chapattis'.

Cinnamon Pancakes

Combine in a large bowl:
¼ cup almond flour
¼ cup arrowroot starch
½ cup chickpea flour
¼ teaspoon baking soda
1/8 teaspoon salt
1 teaspoon cinnamon powder
1 teaspoon cream of tartar

Blend together:
1 Tablespoons lemon juice
1 Tablespoon light oil
1 Tablespoon agave nectar
¾ cup water

Whisk liquid into flour. Mix until smooth. Heat frying pan on medium high. Spoon batter into rounds into the pan. Let cook until bubbles appear on top. Turn over and brown on under side. Serve warm.

Chapter Seven
Remembering Nuts and Seeds

As a fundraiser, our swim team sold bags of peanuts in the shell at the yearly Pan American parade. At the end of the day, my father bought all the remaining bags of peanuts and the family enjoyed cracking and eating peanuts around the kitchen table.

Every autumn, a bowl of mixed nuts with a couple of nut crackers appeared on the living room table. It was always a challenge to see if you could crack a walnut with just the right strength to open it without leaving it in crumbs.

Hazelnuts would routinely go flying because their round little bodies easily evaded the teeth of the nutcracker. As for Brazil nuts, forget it. My little hands never won a battle with their armored exterior. My favorite nut to crack was the almond. Rarely did I ever cause it to crumble.

Nut Butters

Peanut butter was a staple in my diet – not the stuff made with sugar and oil, just peanuts and salt. Under the influence of my parents, I ate peanut butter on apples, bananas, celery, lettuce and cheese. Lavishing peanut butter on something was not reserved for snacking. It was also used as a light meal, or desert.

Peanut Butter Dip

¼ cup peanut butter
1 Tablespoon water

Mix together until smooth. Add more water for a thinner consistency. Store extra in refrigerator.

My lunch for school was a peanut butter and honey sandwich on whole wheat bread. I tried to be food conscious and have an apple for lunch; but without the peanut butter, it just was not the same.

I was introduced to sesame butter, called tahini, through this dip.

Miso Tahini Dip

¼ cup tahini, sesame seed butter
1 teaspoon miso paste
Water

Mix tahini and miso together. Add water to create a thick but runny consistency. Use as a vegetable dip or a sauce over vegetables or noodles.

The dip increased the possibilities of eating raw vegetables. As a child, I ate some vegetables because they tasted good and some vegetables because they tasted good and some I ate just as filler. This dip allowed those vegetables to at least taste good. I found a recipe for tahini in a breakfast muesli recipe in a cookbook for runners. I made Apple Muesli by the quart and ate it for any occasion.

Apple Muesli

Place in the blender:
1 Tablespoon raw oatmeal, soaked in 2 Tablespoons of water for 5 minutes
1 teaspoon honey
1 teaspoon lemon juice
2 teaspoons tahini
1 apple, cored and chopped

Blend until smooth and top with:
1 Tablespoon almond meal
1 Tablespoon tahini

Serve immediately.

I ate just as filler. This dip allowed those vegetables to at least taste good. I found a recipe for tahini in a breakfast muesli recipe in a cookbook for runners. I made Apple Muesli by the quart and ate it for any occasion.

Soaking

Nuts and seeds have an amazing energy potential. With a little water and soil, seeds form into bushes and trees.

Add that potential to your diet and you not only have a great taste but the energy effect charges your body.

The raw food diet capitalizes on this energy because it recommends soaking nuts, seeds, grains and beans before using them. Soaking nuts and seeds unleashes this growing power and aids digestion.

Use raw nuts and seeds for soaking. The larger, dense nuts, like almonds, need 8 hours of soaking while pine nuts do well with 30 minutes. When nuts and seeds are soaked, they become less oily and have a creamy texture when blended. Cashews and macadamia nuts make excellent creamy bases for dips and dressings.

Herb Dip

¾ cup cashews, soaked overnight and drained
½ cup water
1 teaspoon lemon juice
1 teaspoon parsley, chopped
1 teaspoon oregano, chopped
1 teaspoon rosemary, chopped
¼ teaspoon salt

Blend until smooth. Adjust water for thicker consistency. Refrigerate. Best if made the previous day.

Other ways of using soaked nuts are in smoothies and pureed soups to make them rich and creamy. Soaked nuts are only good for a couple days. If you choose to make large batches, consider storing them in the freezer. If you usually only use a certain amount, measure the nuts into separate containers for easy use.

Dehydrating

I prefer dehydrating nuts as a way of preserving them instead of using the freezer for the soaked nuts. After dehydrating, I keep them in the refrigerator to prolong their freshness.

I tend to dehydrate 1-2 pounds of nuts at a time. And even though I have the best of intentions to eat them right away, sometimes I get side tracked on other food. The refrigerator helps prevent the nuts from becoming rancid. However, the refrigerator will not keep things forever. After two months, smell the nuts. If they smell like the refrigerator, compost them and make yourself a fresh batch when you are in the mood for the nuts.

Dehydrated nuts have a wonderful crunchy texture. But do not hesitate to soak them again to soften them if you need a soft nut. Remember the original soaking was to breakdown the enzyme for better digestion. The second soaking can take less time because you are just trying to soften the nuts.

Dehydrating Nuts

1-2 pounds raw nuts, almonds, walnuts or pecans
3 inches kombu seaweed, (optional)
Soaking water

In a bowl, cover nuts and kombu with water. Let stand for 8 hours. Discard kombu. Rinse nuts thoroughly. Place nuts on dehydrator racks and put in dehydrator. Dehydrate for 3 hours on 145°F. Reduce temperature to 115°F and dehydrate until nuts are crunchy, about 12 – 24 hours. Store in an airtight container.

Fruit and spices can be added to the nuts to make granola.

Coconut Granola

1/3 cup raw almonds, soaked for 8 hours
1/3 cup raw walnuts, soaked for 8 hours
1/3 cup raw pumpkin seeds, soaked for 8 hours
1/3 cup raw sunflower seeds, soaked for 8 hours
1/3 cup raisins, soaked for 20 minutes
1/3 cup dates, soaked for 20 minutes
1/3 cup dried coconut, soaked for 20 minutes, (or fresh young coconut)

Rinse nuts and seeds. Strain fruit and reserve juice. Add nut mixture and fruit mixture to food processor. Add in:
1 pear, cored and chopped
¾ teaspoon cinnamon
¾ teaspoon salt

Process until finely chopped. Put on solid dehydrator sheets and dehydrate on 115°F until crunchy, about 12 hours. Store in airtight container. Eat plain as a snack or as a cereal with nut milk.

Toasting

Freshly toasted pine nuts or pumpkin seeds bring a

depth to a salad or a soup, not only in looks but in the

complexity of the nut oil mixing with the vegetables.

Lightly toasting is a process of using heat to release oil from the seed. This gives the seeds an aroma and slightly toasted flavor.

Using a warm, dry frying pan, add nuts or seeds and stir continuously until you smell their nutty aroma. At this point, remove them from the pan even though they do not look toasted. If you wait until they have browned, the seeds are burnt which adds a heavy, burnt flavor your dish. There are times when you want that heavy flavor and there are times when you want the freshness of the seed.

Pine nuts, pumpkin seeds, sunflower seeds and sesame seeds are good for toasting.

Toasted sesame seeds work well over rice and in stir fried vegetables.

Toasted Pine Nuts

Heat frying pan over medium heat. Add
¼ cup pine nuts

Stir constantly for 30 seconds to 1 minute until you can
smell the aroma of the nut. Remove from pan
immediately.

Roasting

Roasting nuts is done in an oven heated to 400°F. You

can flavor the nuts with oil and spices for a crunchy snack or

topping.

Sugar Nuts

Preheat oven to 400°F.

4 cups raw walnuts or pecans
2 Tablespoons butter
¼ cup brown sugar or evaporated sugar cane juice

In a sauce pan, dissolve sugar in butter over medium heat.
Pour over nuts and stir to coat them well. Place nuts on a
cooking sheet in one layer. Bake in oven for 15 to 20
minutes. Stir often. When nuts are golden brown remove
from oven and let cool. Store in airtight container.

One way of not wasting any parts of a squash is to roast

the seeds and use them later for snacking, or added to salads.

Roasted Pumpkin Seeds

Clean and rinse:
Seeds from a squash or pumpkin

Let soak in a bowl for 4 hours in:
Water that covers the seeds
½ teaspoon salt

Preheat oven to 400°F. Drain and rinse seeds. Spread
seeds on a baking sheet into a single layer. Place in warm
oven. Stir seeds after 10 minutes. Roast for 20 minutes
until seeds are slightly brown. Lightly salt and let cool.
Store in an airtight container.

Flour

Nut meal or nut flour is becoming a common

ingredient. You can buy almond flour or you can make it with

your blender. Just make sure that your blender is dry and that

you do not over blend. As soon as the nuts as ground into a

fine powder, stop blending. If you wait, you may have nut butter instead.

Almond flour can be used alone for some recipes that do not require gluten to rise. Almond flour can also be used to substitute a ½ cup of flour in a recipe to give it a little change.

It is also good to have almonds on hand to be able to quickly make some almond flour when you run out of grain flour in the middle of preparing a spur of the moment dish with less than the recommended amounts.

Almond Crust

2 cups almonds, raw or dehydrated
2 - 6 Medjool dates, pitted

In a food processor, add ingredients and pulse process until mixture is coarsely ground. Press into 9-inch dish. Crust is ready to use for no bake or baked recipe. With baking, add prepared filling and bake according to recipe. For a sweeter crust, use more dates.

Milk

When water is just not enough, nut milk gives a dish or a drink some substance. Nut and seeds can give you a variety of nut milks.

Basic Nut Milk

1 cup raw almonds, soak for 8 hours, drained and rinsed
3 cup water

Blend on high until smooth. Pour through a cheese cloth. Squeeze pulp to remove all the water. Discard pulp. Store in refrigerator.

The following are possible substitutions.

- Almond
- Cashew
- Coconut
- Hazelnut
- Walnut
- Chia seed
- Flaxseed
- Hemp
- Quinoa
- Sesame
- Sunflower

If you are short on time and milk or want to make instant milk for a smoothie, blend ¼ cup raw almonds with 1 cup of water. You can then use the cheese cloth to remove the pulp or leave the milk as is and use it.

I prefer homemade nut milk to store bought because many people are sensitive to the binders and gums that are used to thick the store bought variety.

Chopped or Whole

If you find you have no idea how to incorporate nuts and seeds into a recipe, use a small amount to garnish the top of a dish. Chop the large and hard nuts into smaller pieces and leave the smaller softer ones whole.

My parents would add a teaspoon or two of pine nuts and pumpkin seeds while cooking their oatmeal. If I think a soup is going to be a boring mush, I add a handful of chopped walnuts while it is cooking to give it a little texture.

Chapter Eight
Playing with Noodles

My favorite food as an undergraduate in college was spaghetti with red sauce. My sister and I would cook a pound of spaghetti noodles. I would eat a plateful or two with red sauce; and as we were clearing the table, we would snack on the remaining plain noodles straight out of the pan.

Noodles are a wonderful addition to a meal. I think rice and potatoes are great additions to vegetables also but noodles make a meal fun.

Every country has their variation on noodles. In Germany, their noodle is called Spaetzli. In Japan, they have Udon, Soba, and Konjak yam noodles. Bean Thread, Ramen and Lo Mein are the common ones we think of from China but they have many more. Italy began its venture into noodles and pasta during Marco Polo's time when he brought the noodle back from China.

Each noodle lends itself to a different recipe or style of preparation. For instance, it is rare to see an Udon noodle without broth. However, soba noodles can be warm or cold and found in a broth or standing alone. As for Konjak yam noodles, in Japan they were always used in a broth simmered with meat and vegetables.

But do not let the usual styles of preparing noodles hinder you. Depending on the texture and depending on what sauces you like, you can use any noodle you are in the mood for as long as it makes your taste buds and belly happy. The ingredients of noodles vary.

- Wheat
- Buckwheat
- Corn
- Quinoa
- Rice
- Yam – Konjak or Purple yam
- Mung bean
- Vegetables
- Kelp

If you are gluten intolerant or prefer not to eat grain, your best options are noodles made from yam, bean, kelp and vegetables. If pasta is what you are craving, then the grain pastas, with or without gluten will give you a variety of pasta shapes.

Since variety can sometimes lead to waste, I tend to use noodles instead of pasta. I use them either long or broken into pieces depending on the effect I want.

When you have the desire to eat noodles, you only need to think of a few things.

- On the side?
- Cooked together?
- Used as a bed?
- Plain?
- With vegetables?
- Cold or hot?

Bean Thread or Purple Yam

The bean thread and yam noodles are completely cooked when you get them. You only need to rehydrate them.

I use a standard method for preparing the basic noodle. Bring a pot of water to boil, add the noodles, cover and remove from heat. Let the noodles rehydrate for 10 minutes. Drain. The noodles are now ready to be eaten plain or used in a dish.

Bean Thread or Purple Yam Noodle

Bring to boil:
5 cups water or broth

Add in 1-2 serving portions of noodles. Cover.

Remove pan from heat. Let stand for 10 minutes. Drain noodles.
Serve warm or room temperature.

These noodles are good but when they are cooked in a vegetable broth they become outstanding. My favorite broth to soak them in is from greens. After boiling greens, I save the water, then store it in the refrigerator or freezer. When I am ready for noodles, I thaw the broth and use it for the noodles.

If I do not have enough broth, I add plain water.

When the noodles are cooked, add oil and salt or your

favorite sauce.

Spicy Sesame Noodles

In a large bowl, stir until coated:
4 serving cooked spaghetti noodles
2 Tablespoons sesame oil

In a bowl mix until smooth:
1-inch ginger, grated
¼ cup almond butter
¼ cup soy sauce
2 Tablespoons rice vinegar
¼ teaspoon crushed red pepper - optional

In a large bowl, combine noodle and sauce. Serve warm or at
room temperature.

A vegetable stir fry with the bean thread noodles

makes a good lunch. Or you can add either of these noodles

to a soup. In this case, add the noodle just before serving.

These noodles continue to absorb moisture so they will get

wider the longer they are in the broth.

When the noodles are refrigerated they become stiff. To soften and reheat them, add them to boiling water. Turn off burner and let them stand in the water for 1-2 minutes. Drain and they are ready to be eaten.

Konjak

Konjak noodles are made from a yam. They are packed in water that has a seaweed smell to it. A good rinsing will remove most of the odor. These noodles are already cooked so it is a matter of warming them before eating.

However, these noodles are filled with water and tend to leak water. Because of this, you will want to "dehydrate" them before eating. Dry them out using the stove top method discussed in Chapter 5, *Kitchen Tools*.

Heat a skillet on high and add 1-2 tablespoon of oil. The oil prevents the noodles from getting too dry and thus making them chewy. Add the noodles, stirring often. Sauté for 10-15 minutes until there is no water seeping from the noodles. Top with your favorite sauce or use them as an accompaniment to another dish.

Kelp Noodles

Kelp noodles are made from kelp seaweed. They are crunchy and come packed in water. These noodles are used in salads or the basis of salads, and are used in the raw food diet.

You can use a favorite dressing on them or create a sauce.

Eggplant Spaghetti Sauce

In a small bowl, add:
1 Japanese eggplant, peeled, ¼ inch slices
¼ teaspoon salt

Sprinkle salt over eggplant and let sit for 20 minutes. Rinse and drain. Squeeze out excess water. Heat medium size sauce pan, sauté in oil until golden brown: Japanese eggplant

Add in:
¼ cup onions, chopped
¼ cup bell pepper chopped

Cook until tender, then add:
1 glove garlic, crushed
1 Tablespoon oregano
8 ounces tomato sauce
½ cup diced tomatoes
½ cup water
½ teaspoon salt

Simmer for 10 minutes. Add water if sauce gets too thick. Serve warm.

Beet Sauce

In a sauce pan, bring to a boil:
1 small beet, peeled, cut in 1 inch pieces
1 large carrot, peeled, cut in 1 inch pieces
3-inch piece kombu seaweed
1-quart water

Cook on low heat until vegetables as soft. Reserve cooking water. Discard seaweed. In a food processor add:
Cooked vegetables
1 Tablespoon oregano, fresh
¼ teaspoon salt
1 Tablespoon oil
3 Tablespoons of cooking water
Process until smooth. Serve warm.

Vegetables Noodles

Vegetable noodles are vegetables that resemble noodles by the way they are cut.

A spiralizer is a cutter tool that cuts the vegetable as it turns it. This creates long threads of vegetables that resemble a noodle.

The following vegetables make good noodles because of their density:

- Butternut squash
- Daikon radish
- Rutabaga
- Sweet potato
- Turnip
- Zucchini

You may not consider eating a sweet potato raw, but when it is spiralized it has a lighter feeling and mixes well with other vegetables, so there is not one overwhelming flavor. Sometimes thickly cut vegetables get boring because each bite is either all vegetable or all sauce. These noodles allow you to have the perfect blend of both.

Italian Noodles

Put in a bowl:
2 yellow crook neck squash, washed and spiralized
1 small tomato, cut into small bite size pieces
5 olives, cut in half
1 Tablespoon pine nuts

Mix together in a small bowl:
1 Tablespoon oil
1 tablespoon vinegar
2 teaspoons oregano, fresh, chopped
¼ teaspoon salt
Pepper to taste

Combine dressing with squash mixture. Serve.

You can put any of your favorite sauces over vegetable noodles from a tomato sauce to a nut sauce. Or you can add them to a salad. You can create a medley of flavors by combining more than one vegetable and creating a noodle salad.

If you want a crunchier version of any of the vegetable noodles, dehydrate them or quick stir-fry them. In a very hot pan with a little oil, stir noodles until they become slightly stiff. Remove them from the pan and add salt and pepper to taste. You can use these noodles as a snack or add them to a salad. Raw zucchini is a great substitute. It resembles linguini noodles when sliced lengthwise using a vegetable peeler.

For a wider noodle, use a mandolin or knife and cut thin slices length-wise. These slices of zucchini resemble the wide lasagna noodles. Add a cheese, pesto or a red sauce, and you have a light "pasta" meal.

Zucchini Lasagna

2 zucchinis, washed and thinly sliced, length-wise
½ cup cashew cheese
½ cup pesto

Spread 1 slice of zucchini with cashew cheese. Top with 1 slice of zucchini. Spread layer of pesto. Top with 1 slice of zucchini. Spread a layer of cashew cheese. Top with zucchini. Spread a layer of pesto sauce. Start a new stack and follow the same layering until all the zucchini slices are used. Serve at room temperature.

Cashew Cheese

1 cup raw cashews, soaked overnight

Drain and rinse nuts. Process in a food processor until smooth.
Stir together:
Processed cashews
1 Tablespoon rosemary, fresh chopped finely
1 Tablespoon lemon juice
½ teaspoon salt

Best made the day before using.

Pesto

2 cups basil, fresh
¼ cup pine nuts
1 clove garlic
1 teaspoon salt
¼ cup olive oil

Process all ingredients except for the olive oil in a food processor until coarsely chopped. Then drizzle in the olive oil and process until smooth.

Spaghetti Squash

This squash got its name because when cooked, its pulp pulls apart into strands that resemble noodles. The secret is using a fork to remove the pulp in a scraping motion.

Treat spaghetti squash the same as other squashes. Preheat the oven to 350°F. Cut squash open lengthwise and scoop out the seeds. Lay the halves of squash on a baking sheet cut side down. This will allow the squash to cook without becoming dry.

One variation to baking the squash is to put it in a baking dish after it is cut. Add a half cup of vegetable broth or white wine. Cover dish and put in the oven to bake for 30 minutes or so depending on the size of the squash.

Spaghetti Squash

Preheat oven to 350°F.
1 spaghetti squash, cut lengthwise and remove seeds

Put squash, open sides down, on a baking sheet and bake in the oven for 30 – 60 minutes depending on the size of the squash. When a fork easily pierces the pulp, the squash is cooked. Scrape pulp into a bowl using a fork.

Add:
1 Tablespoon oregano, fresh, chopped
I Tablespoon olive oil
½ teaspoon salt

Mix together and serve.

Spaghetti squash can be used as a side dish. It can be eaten by itself or with other vegetables and spices creating a casserole dish.

Twice Baked Spaghetti Squash

Preheat oven to 350°F. 1 spaghetti squash cut lengthwise and remove seeds
Put squash, open sides down, on a baking sheet and bake in the oven for 30 – 60 minutes. When a fork easily pierces the pulp, the squash is done. With a fork scrape pulp into a bowl, set aside.

In a pan, sauté until tender:
¼ cup bell pepper, chopped
½ cup mushrooms, chopped

Stir in:
1 ½ cup tomato sauce
¼ cup sliced black olives
1 Tablespoon oregano, fresh, chopped
2 Tablespoons olive oil
½ teaspoon salt

Cover and cook for 5 minutes. Combine spaghetti squash and sauce and put into a casserole dish. Cover and bake for 20 minutes at 350°F. Serve warm.

Chapter Nine
Simplicity of Soup

Of all the soups my mother made, these three stood out: vegetable soup, split pea soup and gazpacho soup. The first two were eaten warm; the third one was a cold soup.

<u>Gazpacho Soup</u>

1 cucumber, peeled, quartered, deseeded, cut into ¼ inch slices
2 cups tomatoes, peeled and chopped
¼ colored bell pepper, chopped
3 cups tomato juice
¼ cup parsley, chopped fine
1 teaspoon tarragon, dried
1 teaspoon basil, dried
1/8 teaspoon cayenne pepper
½ teaspoon salt

Combine all ingredients in a bowl. Let soup stand for 1 hour before eating. Can be cooled or eaten at room temperature.

When I began to watch how she made soup, I realized there was little mystery to the process. A soup contains solids, liquid and spices.

One day I looked in the refrigerator at all the vegetables. I looked in the cupboard and found several cans of gourmet items bought with good intentions but which we never took the time to use.

I then looked at the overflowing spice rack and suddenly got tired of all the excess stuff we had accumulated for meals that were abandoned before they were made or the left over ingredients of meals that required far less than the minimum amount we could purchase.

Instead of adding to the compost pile, I decided to make a soup. It would either taste good and I would eat it, or the compost would get it but only after I had a little fun.

My first decision was to use a pressure cooker. If I was going to be creative, I wanted to see my results quickly. The vegetable soup my mother made was cooked under pressure for 3 minutes. I decided 3 minutes would be the rule for my soup.

I think my first soup contained beets and chestnuts. I believe the spices were sweet and aromatic, probably something you would find in Indian cuisine, like the Star of Anise.

It was a good try but not to my liking. The flavors did not blend well. I also made too much and got tired of eating it.

Beet Soup

1 beet, medium size, peeled, cubed
1 sweet potato, peeled, cubed
1 stalk celery, chopped
1 bay leaf
1 cup water
3 inches kombu seaweed
¼ teaspoon black pepper ground

Place all ingredients in pressure cooker. Cook under pressure for 3 minutes. Release pressure and open lid. Discard bay leaf and kombu. Add salt as desired. Serve warm.

I kept making soups. There was still a pantry of odds and ends that needed to be used or tossed. With the amount of items on hand, I knew eventually I get the idea of building a soup, one that I enjoyed.

Quickly, I understood that even with the same ingredients, each batch of soup would be different. It was all in the proportions.

I tend not to use measuring cups and spoons. I look to see what I have more of and then base the soup around that vegetable or a specific spice. This gives my soups a theme to the flavor.

Stock

Soups can be either thick or thin depending on the amount of liquid you put in during cooking.

The liquid you use can be plain water or stock - a liquid made from food items.

When you use water alone, the flavors of the vegetables flavor the water. The broth becomes an extension of the vegetables you are eating.

If you use stock, you insert flavors into your soup without adding extra ingredients.

A stock can be made from vegetable or animal products. Most stocks can be purchased either as a concentrate or in liquid form. Some popular types are mushroom, vegetable, kombu seaweed, fish, chicken, or beef.

I prefer water to stock because I do not use onions or garlic in my cooking, which are often used in store bought stock. However, I do reserve the liquid from boiled or steamed vegetables. The liquid can be used repeatedly for boiling or steaming, just add more water. Reserve the leftover water in the refrigerator. This flavored water is your stock when you are ready to make a soup.

Whether I have vegetable stock or not, I add kombu (kelp) seaweed to every soup. I use a 3-inch piece for as much as 2 quarts of soup. If I make a larger batch, I will add a second or third piece depending on the richness of the stock I want.

Parsnip Soup

3 parsnips, peeled, quartered, cut into ½ inch chunks
1 stalk celery, thinly sliced
3 inches kombu seaweed
¼ teaspoon cumin seeds
1/8 teaspoon cayenne pepper
1 ½ cups water or stock

Place ingredients in a large pan. Bring to a boil.
Simmer until parsnips are soft. Discard kombu. Add
salt as desired. Can be pureed. Serve warm.

You might think kombu makes the food taste fishy but it does not. It adds a minerals and potassium which allows me to use less salt overall. In Japan, in place of the common fish stock, kombu stock is used for vegetarian dishes.

I then look at adding mushrooms. Mushrooms give a beefy kind of flavor to the soup. Do I want a light soup or more hearty tasting soup? If you like the flavor of mushrooms but not the texture, leave the mushrooms whole and remove them when your soup is done; or puree them with a little water until they are smooth, then add them to the soup pot for cooking.

Ingredients

Soup can be made from vegetables, beans, noodles, grain; or a combination of ingredients. When deciding what vegetables to put in your soup, here are a few ways to group vegetables.

- Root vegetables
- Summer vegetables
- Leafy greens
- Selection according to a balanced meal in Chapter 2
- Refrigerator selection – whatever you have on hand

Unless you are making a beet borsch soup or want a red soup, I would avoid cooking the soup with red beets. If you want beets in your soup, you can cook them separately, slice them into bite size pieces, and add them as a garnish to your soup bowl just before eating.

If you want more than just vegetables add a handful of beans, rice, nuts and/or noodles. But you can also make your soup mostly beans or grain.

In Japan, when a person is sick, rice soup is eaten to give nourishment without having the stomach work too hard. Sometimes, little pieces of vegetables are added to vary its flavor. The same can be done with beans – a little celery or carrot, or maybe some bell pepper. It is the amount of water that determines whether you have a bowl of beans or bean soup. A lot of water turns a bowl of beans into a soup.

Basic soup

To create your own soup, start with water or stock.

- Two cups of water to make a soup
- 1 cup of water to make a stew

Add three to five cups of vegetables. Pressure cook your soup

for 3 minutes. This will create a soup for 1 or 2 people.

Basic Soup

Put into pressure cooker:
1-2 cups water or broth
3 inches kombu seaweed
3-5 cups vegetables, cut into bite size pieces
1-2 teaspoons spices or dries herbs or
1-2 Tablespoon fresh herbs or
4-8 sprigs of fresh herbs, laid on top of vegetables

Cook under pressure for three minutes. Release pressure
and remove lid. Discard kombu and stems of herbs. Stir
in:
½ teaspoon salt
2 Tablespoons oil

Serve warm.

If you want vegetable soup with beans, use ¼ cup of dried beans that have been soaked for 8 hours. Increase the water amount by ½ cup. Cook the beans for the length of time suggested, minus three minutes. When the beans are cooked, I add the vegetables and pressure cook for the remaining 3 minutes.

To make a vegetable soup with grain, use a ¼ cup of grain and put directly in the pot with the vegetables. Increase your water amount by ½ cup.

If you are interested in noodles in your soup, read the back of the package and make a half serving of noodles according to the package. When the soup is cooked, stir in the noodles to the pot.

Adding spice

When you have determined your basic ingredients, it is time to consider adding herbs and spices.

You can keep the soup simple by adding salt and 2 tablespoons of oil when the soup has finished cooking. Or you can add various herbs or spices.

Use 1-2 teaspoons of dried spices. Use 1-3 tablespoons of fresh herbs. With the fresh herbs, you can leave them on their stems.

I use several stems of herbs and lay them on the top of the vegetables before I close the lid for cooking. When the soup is cooked, I remove the stems. Some of the leaves will have separated from the stem. I leave those in the soup. This allows the flavor of the soup to maintain a certain level of spice intensity. If I left the large bundle of herbs in the soup, the flavor of the herb would overpower the flavor of the vegetables.

Thickening the broth

For a thicker broth, use starchy vegetables, like potatoes, parsnips and sweet potatoes. If the vegetables do not break up in cooking, mash a portion of the vegetables or puree a third of the soup and mix it back in the pot.

Pureeing changes the flavor of a soup. It mellows and harmonizes it. Pureed soup is one method of taking soup you may not appreciate and making it taste good. It also is a good way to consume vegetables that otherwise you might not eat.

When I am unfamiliar with a vegetable, I do two things. I use a small amount in a recipe; and keep the pieces big enough so that it does not show up in every spoonful. It also makes it easy to pick out if I really do not care for the taste of it.

To create a creamy broth, use rice, lentils and nut butters. Start cooking the rice and lentils first so that they completely breakdown in the time it takes to cook the vegetables. This allows the rice and lentils to turn to mush but keep the vegetables tender and formed. If the grain or beans are not completely broken down when the vegetables are finished cooking, they will break down when you add the salt and stir to mix everything together.

You can also use nuts for a creamy consistency. Whole nuts can be blended with some of the broth and returned to the soup. Or you can mix some of the broth with 2 tablespoons of nut butter.

Chapter Ten
Salads with Character

My mother's idea of a dinner from her childhood was an animal protein, a salad, a cooked vegetable, and a starch. This meant that at least once a day, we would have a salad as part of the meal. A variety of dressings would be available on the table so each one of us could flavor the salad to our liking.

At one point we acquired the Salad Master which sliced and shredded vegetables into an array of shapes and sizes. With this tool and a book on eating raw food from Norman Walker, we expanded our use of fresh vegetables.

Our salads of iceberg lettuce and cucumber were transformed into works of art. We started eating a Waldorf salad, and if apricots were ripe on the tree, we would add those to the fruit salad; or we might have a salad served on individual plates.

Rainbow Salad

5 leaves red leaf lettuce
¼ cup raw beet finely grated
¼ cup carrot finely grated
¼ cup chopped celery
1 sliced of apple
Lay lettuce on plate. Arrange each vegetable on a different area of the plate.

Mix together:
¼ cup of plain yogurt
Honey to taste
Pinch of salt

Pour over salad and serve.

Salads can be made of fruit or vegetables or a combination of the two. There are noodle salads, bean salads, and grain salads like the one that is made with bulgur wheat. Some salads are cooked; some are raw; and some are a combination of the two.

For this section, I will deal with fruit and vegetables salads.

Fruit Salads

Eating fruit salads can be refreshing and light. They are good for breakfast, a light meal, or an evening snack.

The best way to make a fruit salad is to start with the fruits that are in season locally. This will give you the sweetest fruit possible. Cut fruit into small bite size pieces. Adding a soft fruit, like an apricot, with a hard fruit, Japanese persimmon, can make the chewing easier.

Waldorf Salad

1 apple, chopped into small bite size pieces
1 stalk celery, cut into ¼ inch pieces
¼ walnuts, chopped coarsely

Mix together in a bowl and serve.

Fruit combination options:

- Northern fruit – apples, berries, cherries, loquats, peaches, pears, persimmons
- Southern fruit – banana, mango, papaya, coconut
- Citrus only – orange, grapefruit, kumquats
- Or a little of each

You can mix in some nuts – chopped almonds, walnuts or hazelnuts, for a crunch; or chopped dried fruit – raisins, figs, coconut, or dates, for a concentrated sweet.

For sauce ideas:

Depending on the fruit you use and the amount of moisture in the fruit, simply stirring the fruit will create a juice for the fruit. A variation on the juice is to add a teaspoon of balsamic vinegar for each serving of fruit. Instead of cropped nuts, you can make a nut cream sauce.

Cashew Sauce

1 cup cashew, raw and soaked for 4 hours
1 Medjool date, soak for 20 minutes, reserve soaking water
½ teaspoon lemon juice
½ teaspoon salt

Blend until smooth. Use date soaking water to thin to desired consistency.

Variation: Replace cashew nuts for soaked macadamia nuts.

Alternatively, drizzle nut butter, thinned with water, over the fruit. These butters can be made from sesame seeds, walnuts or almonds.

Vegetable salads

Vegetable salads composed of light vegetables can be used as a side dish or snack, or additions of root vegetables, olives and nuts will transform them into a main dish. Vegetable salads can have one ingredient or a long list of ingredients. They can be all raw or partially cooked.

Building a Salad

The common green salad is made with lettuce as a base.

Types of lettuce include:

- Iceberg
- Romaine
- Green or red leaf
- Spinach, Chard, Kale
- Field greens – radicchio, arugula, kale, dandelion
- Bibb

Chop, shred, or tear these leafy greens into bite size or smaller pieces. Instead of leafy greens, you can build a salad with cabbage:

- Green
- Napa
- Red
- Savoy

Spinach, Chard and Kale have hardier leaves than field greens and are good in wilted salads.

Warm Spinach Salad

In a bowl, mix together:
2 Tablespoon oil
1Tablespoon cider vinegar
¼ teaspoon Dijon mustard
¼ teaspoon salt
Pepper to taste
Set aside.

In a warm non-stick skillet, put 1 Tablespoon raw pine nuts.
Stir until you can smell the aroma of the pine nuts but before
the pine nuts turns golden brown. Remove nuts from skillet.

Add into skillet:
¼ cup sliced mushrooms
Cook for 1 minute. Remove skillet from heat. Stir in:
2 cups spinach leaves
Dressing from above
Stir until leaves are coated. Transfer to a serving bowl and top
with pine nuts. Serve immediately.

Once you have decided whether you are using lettuce

or cabbage, or a combination of the two, it is time to add non-

leafy vegetables.

Some non-leafy vegetable choices:

- Carrot
- Celery
- Radish
- Broccoli
- Summer squash – zucchini, crook neck, patty pan
- Green beans
- Beet
- Bell pepper

<u>Cucumber Cole Slaw</u>

1-inch ginger root, peeled, finely chopped
¼ head of small green cabbage, finely chopped
1 ½ inch piece yellow crook neck squash, coarsely chopped
1 small stalk celery, coarsely chopped
4 inches cucumber, peeled, seeds removed, coarsely chopped

Put ingredients in a large bowl. Toss with
5 small green olives, halved
¼ cup pumpkin seeds
2 Tablespoons oil
2 Tablespoons vinegar
½ teaspoon salt

Serve chilled or at room temperature. Best made a day ahead.

Then consider adding a fruit, such as:

- Tomato
- Avocado
- Olive

Top with nuts, seeds, corn chips or nutritional yeast.

Building Character

Creating character with your salad is accomplished by the way you cut up the vegetables. Whenever possible, I avoid working hard to eat a salad. I keep my salad ingredients small to bite size for ease of chewing.

Some restaurant house salads have chunks of carrot and thick slices of cucumber on top of lettuce pieces that are as big as the palm of my hand. In those instances, I ask for a steak knife and cut the chunks into bite size pieces.

It is not just about the looks

Vegetables have a different flavor depending on how you cut them. You can experiment with this using a carrot. Cut it in a variety of styles.

- Slice it straight across and then on a diagonal.
- Cut it to a length of one inch; then 1/8 inch cuts width-wise; and then cut those flat pieces in 1/8 inch slices. You will have formed "match sticks".
- Grate some carrot coarsely.
- Grate some carrot with a fine grate.
- Finally, chop a piece into irregular shaped small pieces.

Taste each one of the cuts. Some cuts will have a lot of flavor; some will have so little flavor that their effect is simply to add color.

Chunky salads

Some salads are a combination of chunks of vegetables, either parboiled or raw and tossed in a dressing. To parboil a vegetable, bring a pot of water to a boil. Add the bite size

pieces of vegetables and cook until the color of the vegetable

becomes bright.

In the case of broccoli, the color will be a bright green.

This can take 1 – 3 minutes. Remove the vegetables from the

water and cool them in cold water with ice.

Broccoli Salad

2 cups broccoli, cut into small florets
¼ cup red bell pepper finely chopped
2 Tablespoons toasted pine nuts
2 Tablespoons Italian dressing

Bring a large pan of water to boil, add broccoli florets and
cook for 1 minute until broccoli is bright green.

Remove broccoli from water and rinse under cold water to
stop the cooking process. Put broccoli in a large bowl. Mix
in the rest of the ingredients.

Serve cool or at room temperature.

Dressing the salad

The difference in whether one eats a salad is many times the choice of dressing.

<u>Orange Dressing</u>

Wisk together in a bowl:

1/3 cup olive oil
1 Tablespoon rice vinegar
Juice from 1 orange
1 teaspoon Dijon mustard

One family went back for seconds on salad when it was tossed in blue cheese with a hint of teriyaki sauce, and topped with corn chips and avocado.

A traditional Italian husband often eats his salads with just balsamic vinegar, olive oil, salt and pepper.

Avocado Dressing

Blend until smooth:

¼ cup raw cashews, soaked and rinsed
½ cup hot water
2 avocados
2 Medjool dates, seed removed and soaked 20 minutes
½ teaspoon salt

On one family occasion, my sister made a huge bowl of salad. She dressed it with Caesar dressing and added cranberries and toasted pumpkin seeds. It was gobbled up quickly. We all wanted seconds before we even started the main course.

Ginger Vinaigrette

Mix together in a bowl:

3 Tablespoon olive oil
2 Tablespoons apple cider vinegar
1-inch ginger, peeled and minced
½ teaspoon salt

"Cheezy" Vinaigrette

Wisk together in a bowl:
1/3 cup olive oil
2 Tablespoons balsamic vinegar
1 Tablespoon nutritional yeast
1 teaspoon Dijon mustard
¼ teaspoon salt

Hidden Valley Ranch has a great TV commercial. Add

a good dressing, and children as well as adults, will eat their

vegetables.

Pina Colada Dressing

Blend together until smooth:
1/3 cup raw cashews, soaked and drained
1/3 cup coconut butter
¼ cup pineapple juice
1 teaspoon lemon juice
½ teaspoon salt

A few salad dressing ideas:

- Salad dressings tend to have an acid and an oil.

- Common acids are lemon, lime, sour plum and vinegar.

- Common oils are olive, coconut, grape seed, and nut
  oils and nut butters.

- Combine a sour flavor with oil, add salt and pepper
  and you have a salad dressing. If you want it a little
  sweet, add honey, agave nectar, Medjool dates or
  Stevie.

Whisk or blend the ingredients together for a smooth

dressing.

Salads made from fruit or lettuces are best eaten the

same day. Salads made with chunks of vegetables or

cabbages are best made the day before to allow the dressing to

flavor and tenderize the vegetables or cabbage.

Chapter Eleven
Elemental Stir Fry

While studying the Chinese Nutrition course, the instructor explained how he cooked his food. He heated a wok, added a little water, added the vegetables, stirred them around a few times; covered the wok for 1 minute, and his food was done. He would mix in a little sesame oil and the food was ready to eat.

I spoke with my dentist the other day about home cooking. With his wife being Chinese, nightly meals were usually Chinese - a stir fry with rice on the side. The nightly stir fry varied by the available vegetables.

Stir frying is easy. The longest part is preparing the vegetables. I use a non-stick wok. It allows me to use little to no water and to add my oil after cooking. I prefer the taste of uncooked oil. It has a cleaner flavor to me.

Basic Stir Fry

Figuring out what you want to put into a stir fry is the first step. You can keep the ingredients simple in the stir fry and begin by cooking just one vegetable.

You could do asparagus or mushrooms or sugar peas or even just bean sprouts. Or you can include a number of vegetables.

Good stir frying vegetables include:
- Mushrooms
- Zucchini, summer squash
- Bell peppers
- Mung bean or soy sprouts
- Cabbage
- Celery
- Water chestnuts
- Broccoli, Brussels sprouts, kohlrabi
- Bok choy
- Snap peas, snow peas
- Ginger

Stir Fry Combinations

Mushroom, Bell Pepper
**

Bok Choy, Snow Pea, Mung Bean Sprouts
**

Broccoli, Water Chestnut, Ginger
**

Zucchini, Cabbage, Mushroom
**

Asparagus, Mushroom, Bell Pepper, Mung Bean Sprouts
**

Snap Pea, Bell Pepper
**

Brussels Sprouts, Celery, Snap Pea

Allow about 3 cups of raw vegetables per serving. This gives you the option of a large amount t of a few vegetables or small quantities of a variety of vegetables.

Chop or slice your vegetables into bite size pieces. Some vegetables you will keep long, like mung bean sprouts which are close to 2 inches but become soft when cooked, so the size does not matter.

When cutting the vegetables, think about how long they will take to cook. You may make them smaller to decrease their cooking time or keep them large so that they will cook at the same rate as the other vegetables you are using.

Sort the chopped vegetables into piles according to their cooking time. For instance, asparagus will take several minutes longer to cook than bell pepper depending how well cooked you like your food.

Put the denser vegetables into the pan at the beginning of stir frying. This will allow them to become tender along with the more delicate and faster cooking vegetables.

Heat the wok to medium high heat. When the wok is hot, add the first vegetable. Stir the vegetable so it gets evenly cooked. Cook for 1-2 minutes.

Then add the next vegetable and repeat the process until all the vegetables are cooking in the wok.

Some vegetables may take the same amount of time. In this case, add those vegetables together. An example would be when using snap peas, bell pepper and mung bean sprouts which all take the same amount of cooking time.

If you find that the vegetables are not cooked enough for your liking, add 2 tablespoons of water or unsweetened tea, and cover the wok for 2 minutes. Reduce the heat to medium.

When the two minutes are done, uncover and stir the vegetables. If they are still not cooked enough for you, cover and cook for another 2 minutes.

Once the stir fry is cooked, remove it from the heat and add flavoring.

For added flavor, top the stir fried vegetables with one tablespoon of sesame seeds, pumpkin seeds, pine nuts or thinly cut nori seaweed.

Sour and Salty Sauce

2 teaspoons soy sauce
2 teaspoons rice vinegar
2 teaspoons sesame oil

Mix together.

Nothing Fancy Sauce

2 teaspoons olive oil
Salt to taste

Drizzle over vegetables.

Sweet and Sour Sauce

2 teaspoons Mirin wine
2 teaspoons rice vinegar
2 teaspoons olive oil
Salt to taste

Mix together.

Miso Sauce

1 teaspoon miso
1 teaspoon tahini
1 teaspoon vinegar
2 teaspoon water

Stir until smooth.

Creamy and Salty Sauce

2 teaspoons soy sauce
2 teaspoons Earth Balance

Mix into warm vegetables.

Chapter Twelve
Outdoor Grilling

While visiting family in Illinois during the winter, it mattered not whether there was rain, snow, hot or cold weather, this family used the grill. Somehow the idea of grilling in the snow, all bundled up, made this Southern California girl laugh.

However, they were really enjoyed their barbecue meals. Grilling vegetables allows a texture and a taste variation from other types of cooking.

To prepare vegetables for grilling, marinate them overnight or cut them up at the last minute. Then grill them, add some salt and oil when they are done and enjoy.

BBQ Corn on the Cob

Soak the corn with the husks still intake in cold water for 30 minutes. Place on the grill and turn every 2 minutes until the corn is heated on all sides, about 10 minutes. Serve warm.

Grilled Snap Peas

Mix in a bowl and let sit for 1 hour:
2 cups snap peas, washed and strings removed
1 Tablespoon oregano, fresh
1 teaspoon Italian seasoning
¼ teaspoon salt
1 Tablespoon lime juice
1 Tablespoon olive oil

Strain out vegetables from juice. Reserve juice and use if vegetables get dry during grilling. Grill on a solid pan stirring every 2 minutes. Remove when peas are slightly tender. Serve warm.

Grilled Vegetable Medley

Mix in a bowl and let sit for 1 hour:
½ cup mushrooms, quartered
½ cup zucchini, halved and sliced into ¼ inch pieces
½ cup yellow crook neck squash, quartered and sliced into ¼ inch pieces
1 small bell pepper, cut into 1 inch squares
2 Tablespoon oregano, fresh
2 teaspoon Italian seasoning
½ teaspoon salt
2 Tablespoons lemon juice
2 Tablespoons olive oil

Strain vegetables from their juice. Grill on a solid pan stirring every 5 minutes until the vegetables and cooked to your liking, about 10-20 minutes. Serve warm.

Grilled Bell Peppers

1 large red bell pepper

Cut in quarters length-wise. Place on grill. Turn every 2 minutes until peppers are warm but not burnt. Remove from flame. Add salt and pepper to taste. Serve warm.

Chapter Thirteen
Baking and Roasting

The oven became more important in our kitchen when the microwave died years ago. Since the microwave was a glorified warmer, whether that was for food or tea, it never got replaced.

With no access to a microwave, I had to relearn the wonders of the oven. I found it does two jobs: It warms and it cooks.

Warming food

Heat the oven to 350°F. Add the food dishes you want warmed; and in 20 minutes, your meal is ready. If you just want to take the chill off an item, once you put the food into the oven, turn the oven off. In 20 minutes, your food will be pleasantly warm but not overcooked.

Baking

Most vegetables are baked using 350°F. heat. This is a slow-cook method that brings out the sweetness of the vegetable.   Root vegetables become sweeter when baked.

Baked Winter Squash

1 winter squash – butternut, acorn, kabocha, banana

Preheat oven to 350°F. Cut in half. Remove seeds. Lay in a baking pan, cut side down. Bake for 40 minutes to 1 hour or until a fork easily pierces the pulp. Serve warm.

Baked Cauliflower

1 small cauliflower
½ cup white wine
3-inch piece kombu seaweed

Preheat oven to 350°F. Remove outer leaves and wash cauliflower. Place cauliflower stems down, wine, and kombu in baking dish with lid. Cover.

Bake for 20 minutes or until tender. Discard kombu. Serve warm.

Baked Carrots

2 large carrots

Preheat oven to 350°F. Peel carrots. Cut in half. Place in baking dish with lid. Cover. Bake for 30 minutes or until tender. Serve warm.

Roasting

The roasting process cooks vegetables with intense heat. This causes the vegetables to cook on the outside faster than they cook on the inside.

Season vegetables with oil or a combination of herbs and oil, then place in an open baking dish. Preheat oven to 425°F. Cooking time varies depending on the density of the vegetables.

- Root vegetables and winter squash can take 40 minutes to 1 hour to cook.

- Summer squashes can take 20 to 40 minutes to roast.

To determine if your food is cooked, first find out if it is tender. Then does it have a slightly roasted coloring. If food is getting dark but not tender, reduce the oven heat to 350° F. and continue roasting.

Check the progress of the vegetables every 15 minutes. Be sure to stir them at these intervals so that they brown and cook evenly. Stirring also recoats the vegetables with the

seasoning. Add a few tablespoons of water or oil if the

vegetables seem dry.

Roasted Baby Squash and Carrots

Preheat oven to 425°F. Mix together:
6 baby patty pan squash
1 carrot, peeled and diagonally sliced
1 Tablespoon oregano, fresh
Olive oil

Put vegetables in a baking dish and bake in oven. Stir
vegetables every 15 minutes until tender. About 40
minutes. Add salt to flavor. Serve warm.

Roasted Root Vegetables

Preheat oven to 425°F. In a large bowl, mix together:

½ cup butternut squash, peeled, cut into ½ inch cubes
½ cup parsnips, peeled, cut into ½ inch pieces
½ cup kohlrabi, peeled, cut into ½ inch cubes
½ cup golden beet, peeled, cut into ½ inch cubes
2 Tablespoons balsamic vinegar
2 Tablespoons olive oil
½ teaspoon salt
½ teaspoon black pepper, coarsely ground

Transfer to baking dish large enough for vegetables to lie in a single layer on the bottom of the pan. Roast in oven for 40 minutes or until tender, stirring every 15 minutes. Serve warm.

Roasted Sweet Potatoes

Preheat oven to 425°F.
In a large bowl, mix together:

1 cup sweet potato, peeled, cut into ½ inch cubes
1 cup kohlrabi, peeled, cut into ½ inch cubes
½ cup sunchokes, peeled, cut into ½ inch cubes
1 Tablespoon tarragon, fresh, chopped finely
3 Tablespoons olive oil
½ teaspoon salt
½ teaspoon black pepper, coarsely ground

Transfer to baking dish large enough for vegetables to lie in a single layer on the bottom of the pan. Roast in oven for forty minutes or until tender. Stir vegetables every 15 minutes. Serve warm.

Conclusion

With this reintroduction to food, your journey in your kitchen will bring you fun.

You now can see that food can be combined in a variety of ways to bring more vegetables into your diet without an overwhelming list of ingredients.

Look for the simple approach to preparing food and you will enjoy your time in your kitchen. Review the chapters often to get a feel for how certain foods can be prepared then let your imagination free.

Recipe Index

www.ingramcontent.com/pod-product-compliance
Lightning Source LLC
Chambersburg PA
CBHW071354280526
45787CB00001B/322